HYPERTENSION:

EVALUATION AND TREATMENT

Medicines are nothing in themselves if not properly used.
But the very hands of the Gods, if employed with reason and
prudence.

Herophilus, 300 BC

HYPERTENSION:

EVALUATION AND TREATMENT

EDWARD D. FROHLICH, MD, MACP, FACC
Alton Ochsner Distinguished Scientist
Vice President for Academic Affairs
Alton Ochsner Medical Foundation
New Orleans, LA

Professor of Medicine and of Physiology
Louisiana State University School of Medicine

Clinical Professor of Medicine and
Adjunct Professor of Pharmacology
Tulane University School of Medicine

Editor: Jonathan W. Pine, Jr.
Managing Editor: Keith Rhett Murphy
Marketing Manager: Daniell T. Griffin
Production Coordinator: Peter J. Carley
Project Editor: Susan Rockwell
Illustration Planner: Wayne Hubbel
Design Coordinator: Mario Fernandez
Typesetter and Digitized Illustrations: Peirce Graphic Services, Inc.
Printer/Binder: Mack Printing Group

Accurate indications, adverse reactions and dosage schedules for drugs are provided in this book, but it is possible that they may change. The reader is urged to review the package information data of the manufacturers of the medications mentioned.

Printed in the United States of America

Library of Congress Cataloging-in-Publication Data

The publishers have made every effort to trace the copyright holders for borrowed material. If they have inadvertently overlooked any, they will be pleased to make the necessary arrangements at the first opportunity.

To purchase additional copies of this book, call our customer service department at **(800) 638-0672** or fax orders to **(800) 447-8438.** For other book services, including chapter reprints and large quantity sales, ask for the Special Sales department.

Canadian customers should call **(800) 665-1148,** or fax **(800) 665-0103.** For all other calls originating outside of the United States, please call **(410) 528-4223** or fax us at **(410) 528-8550.**

Visit *Williams & Wilkins* on the Internet: http://www.wwilkins.com or contact our customer service department at **custserv@wwilkins.com.** Williams & Wilkins customer service representatives are available from 8:30 am to 6:00 pm, EST, Monday through Friday, for telephone access.

98 99 00
1 2 3 4 5 6 7 8 9 10

Preface

HYPERTENSION: EVALUATION AND TREATMENT continues to be a most timely subject for the practicing physician. While the importance of hypertension as a major clinical problem has been a major focus for many years of the practicing primary care physician, it has drawn perhaps less attention and the more fractionated interest of the more specialized practitioners until more recent years. Thus, hypertension has been of interest to the nephrologist if parenchymal disease of the kidney and renal arterial disease were present. This aspect of the disease is no small share of the problem since, despite reduction in deaths from stroke and coronary heart disease, endstage renal disease continues to increase in numbers of patients afflicted and in unchecked annual healthcare costs (whether in North America, Europe or Japan). The endocrinologist has focused on the patient with an elevated arterial pressure, particularly if there were also problems related to thyroid, adrenal, parathyroid, growth hormone disease, the less common patient with pheochromocytoma and, of course, the tremendous number of patients with the complicating and comorbid disease, diabetes mellitus. The cardiovascular physician's interest, unfortunately, has been more concerned with hypertension as an independent risk of coronary artery disease. This, of course, focused on the problems of left ventricular hypertrophy, sudden cardiac death, congestive heart failure, angina pectoris, accelerated atherosclerosis with complicating myocardial infarction, and with dissecting aneurysm. And, today, congestive heart failure secondary to hypertension is among the most common causes for hospitalization in the United States; and this frequency continues to increase in the elderly. This rather perfunctory and fragmented attention to these problems is best evidenced by the self-assessment and board certifying examinations wherein little emphasis had been devoted to the hypertensive disease and its diagnosis and treatment.

More recently, however, cardiovascular medicine has focused more attention on hypertension and risk factor prevention. The American College of Cardiology has established a standing committee on hypertensive diseases and has included prevention and hypertensive diseases importantly in its recent self-assessment study programs. In part, much of this recent attention can be attributed to the long-awaited recognition of hypertension as a major risk factor underlying the development of coronary heart disease (of the arterioles as well as epicardial arteries) and deaths from coronary heart disease. Recognition and correction of those factors has been appreciated more and more as a preventive measure as well as in the overall wellness and rehabilitative programs for patients with a prior history of myocardial infarction.

Unfortunately, even following the recent Joint National Committee's fifth and sixth reports, too many patients with hypertension remain unrecognized, untreated or treated ineffectively. Moreover, recognition and effective early treatment, designed to prevent premature cardiovascular morbidity and mortality, has become an important necessity of the nation's health care for the new millennium. However, less efforts are still being expended by subspecialty physicians in the recognition of the existence of hypertension and its associated complications. By this I re-emphasize the progression and intrinsic risk associated with left ventricular hypertrophy, *per se,* the importance of arteriolar disease of the coronary circulation, sudden cardiac death,

v

heart failure, acceleration of atherogenesis, and the less appreciated involvement of the renal circulation that leads unrelentingly to end-stage renal disease. Abundant evidence is now available that supports the thesis that these risks are greater among special demographic segments of our population: the black patient, the person with a family history of premature cardiovascular death, patients with carbohydrate intolerance and diabetes mellitus, the elderly individual, men and women with other specific medical problems, those individuals who unwittingly take certain over-the-counter and prescribed drugs that may exacerbate hypertensive disease and, of course, those patients with other coexisting risk factors such as obesity, alcohol and tobacco abuse, and hyperlipidemias.

This monograph was written at the suggestion of my good friend Doctor Willis Hurst who felt that one individual's overview of the foregoing problem may be of value to the physician whose practice is oriented to cardiovascular medicine. To this end, the book is written with this orientation providing a strong hemodynamic and fundamental cardiovascular mechanistic basis for the approach to the hypertensive patient and the effective management of specifically identified categorical populations of patients with hypertension. Nevertheless, this text was designed for the primary care physicians as well as each of the specialized physicians to underscore the necessity to recognize, evaluate and treat all patients with hypertension.

It is not the intent of the book to present an all-encompassing and encyclopedic multiauthor review of every aspect of hypertensive disease and all of the pertinent references that such a text deserves. Rather, as expressed above, the text was written to provide for the cardiovascular, renal, and endocrinologically oriented clinicians as well as generalists and the interested student, with both a clinical, yet fundamental approach to this broad subject. Admittedly, the text is written with the biases of one individual. However, I make every effort to advance generally accepted concepts and, when controversy exists, I identify those areas and qualify the expressed ideas as those drawn from my personal experience, clinically and investigatively. There has been a deliberate intent to exclude distracting references from the flow of the text. However, at the conclusion of each chapter, the reader is provided with a suggested list of reading material that is intended to complement that chapter's message. This list focuses primarily on the author's bibliography in order to provide further rationale and more extensive explanations for his personal overviews. Some of these selected references are very recent, and others are suggested for their overall importance and value to the overall subject.

The background on pathophysiology and pharmacology was included to provide the reader with a necessary fundamental background that should enable the readers to arrive at their own conclusions on the most appropriate treatment plans for groups of patients with essential hypertension. To this end, we hope that this rationale for treatment by one author will not only be of value for meaningful practice today but to facilitate adaptation into newer clinical treatment and management approaches for future medical practice.

Acknowledgments

In 1956, when I began my housestaff training following graduation from medical school, the treatment of hypertension was difficult and hazardous. The rice fruit diet had already been shown to be effective in some patients; patients were carefully referred for lumbo-dorsal sympathectomy or adrenalectomy; the ganglion blocking drugs were being employed by some confident and bold clinicians; and trials with hydralazine, the various alkaloids, and reserpine were in progress. Hospital beds were filled with patients having been admitted with hypertensive emergencies, congestive heart failure resulting from hypertension, dissecting aneurysms, strokes, coronary heart disease and myocardial infarctions. The promise of controlling or preventing glomerulonephritis with early treatment of beta-hemolytic streptococcal infections was only recently established. How fortunate, then, that in one's own professional career, it has become possible to have been able to get a real hold on this problem and to control it.

Yes, in these 40 years deaths from stroke have been diminished by almost 70 percent and, from coronary heart disease, by over 50 percent. Intensive care units have far fewer patients with dissecting aneurysms, and hypertensive emergencies are indeed rarities in stark contrast with the picture of 40 years ago. The era of modern preventive cardiology had been established. Detection and recognition of the patient with hypertension have been emphasized over-and-again, and effective antihypertensive therapy is now possible anywhere in the world. More specifically, in the United States, much credit must be given to the National High Blood Pressure Education Program championed by the National Heart, Lung, and Blood Institute of the National Institutes of Health, professional health oriented organizations, and the research and education programs supported by the National Institutes of Health, the American Heart Association, and the innovative creativity of the pharmaceutical industry.

Over these 40 years it has been my privilege to participate actively and broadly in this success story of medicine—clinically, investigationally, educationally, and organizationally. During these very exciting and professionally rewarding years, I have also been privileged to have had the intellectual and professional support and stimulation by three major figures and colleagues in this story. Dr. Irvine Heinly Page was among the first in the world to emphasize the nature of hypertensive disease. His fundamental and clinical accomplishments are legend in this story of conquest of disease from the discovery and peptide sequencing of angiotensin II and the elaboration of the renopressor system, to the discovery of serotonin, the description of resetting baroreceptor function in hypertension, to the unique concept of the multifactorial nature of hypertension through his elucidation of his mosaic of hypertension. Dr. Edward David Freis was the first to conceive of and to establish a multicenter, placebo-controlled study that clearly demonstrated the safety and efficacy of antihypertensive therapy not only in controlling arterial pressure but in reducing morbidity and mortality. This series of the landmark Veterans Administration Cooperative Study reports has become a classical accomplishment in the history of medicine, and he has received his just credits for organizing and insuring the scientific conduct of these long-term studies (which continue to this date). However, less known have been his fundamental and important clinical and laboratory studies that were concerned with the pathophysiology of hypertensive cardiac and vascular disease. The third, and by no means a lesser leader in hypertension with whom I have enjoyed a close personal and professional relationship, is Dr. Harriet Pearson Dustan, a tireless worker in the multiple vineyards of hypertension research and treatment. She has been a major force in our society—through public, volunteer, and professional organizations, as well as in the educational and research spheres—in placing hypertension in the proper perspective for the National Heart, Lung and Blood Institute; Institute of Medicine; American Heart Association; and the American College of Physicians. Her interests have exceeded those of research and patient care and have impacted importantly on other difficult avenues of concern: ethics, medico-social responsibility, and education for the professional as well as lay person. In my admittedly biased (but, I am certain, broadly agreed) point of view, without the vigorous efforts of these three giants, medicine would not have reaped the benefits of our clinical and scientific achievements as rapidly. We (and certainly I) owe much to these outstanding physicians, scientists, and human beings and friends. Working and knowing these individuals has been a genuine professional joy in my life.

On a more personal note, I wish to express my appreciation and deep satisfaction to my many patients over these years. Through my clinical experience and my personal relationships with them I have learned much about hypertensive disease. These clinical experiences have continuously stimulated an ongoing flow of questions which have precipitated four decades of clinical and more fundamental research. It has been these research experiences which have provided the rewards to many others as well as myself in seeing improved clinical outcomes, less morbidity and reduced mortality from hypertensive disease and its complications. Similarly, I wish to express my deepest appreciation to the many professional colleagues and clinical and laboratory research fellows who volunteered to spend two or more years of their lives in my fundamental and clinical research laboratories. Our work together continues to provide the excitement, fuel, and drive to explore new knowledge, increasing insight into hypertensive disease and therapeutic mechanisms, and ongoing conviction to the long-standing credo of clinical investigators. Yes, patient care, investigation, and teaching are the professional life-sustaining activities and lifeblood of the clinical investigator that makes an academic life so fulfilling.

It goes without saying that none of the foregoing human relationships and experiences would have been possible without a deep and warm relationship with family. It was my parents, early on in my life, that instilled into me a love and respect for education and a deep commitment for humane considerations. I am ever-grateful and always consciously aware and thankful to my loving wife Sherry who has helped to keep me focused on what is truly important in life—respect for human welfare; the need for personal communication with patients, colleagues, and friends; the necessity of a caring professional demeanor and an abiding concern for the quality of life of those who are unwell. Without her support and encouragement and that of my children, Margie, Bruce and Lara, my academic career would not have been possible. They fully understood that which is required for a professional and academic life, the long hours away from home and longer hours away from their company while working undisturbed at my desk at home.

I want to express my warm appreciation to my office staff and, especially, my assistant, Mrs. Caramia Fairchild, who has conscientiously and meticulously worried through my manuscripts, copy editing, and relationships with my publishers. I also thank Gene Kearn, of Igaku-Shoin Publishers, and Jonathan Pine, Keith Murphy and Pete Carley of Williams & Wilkins for their support in this textbook. Putting together a multiauthor textbook is an arduous task, and Gene was most helpful in my efforts with such a volume a number of years ago. But, I have learned that a single-author textbook (such as this) is fraught with many more different and formidable issues. I am grateful to him, too, for his contribution. Jonathan, Keith and Pete helped me greatly when Williams & Wilkins assumed responsibility for this work when that publisher acquired Igaku-Shoin of this country.

Finally, I am truly grateful to you who are reading these words. For without your individual and personal interest and desire to translate these words into clinical experience, to transfer my thoughts and experiences to your possible practice is what makes this work worthwhile. In the final analysis, this is what must be fundamental to writing this or any other book.

Contents

SECTION I

PATHOPHYSIOLOGY AND CLINICAL EVALUATION

Chapter 1

Pathophysiology:
Disease Mechanisms

Systemic arterial hypertension is one of the most common cardiovascular diseases of industrialized populations. It affects approximately 20 percent of adults in these societies, and even a higher proportion in certain demographic groups (e.g., blacks, elderly). The disease is a major treatable risk factor (Table 1.1) underlying coronary heart disease, and it exacerbates and accelerates the atherosclerotic process. Hypertension is therefore a key determinant of risk for premature cardiovascular morbidity and mortality associated with major cardiac disorders including small arteriolar disease of the coronary circulation, occlusive epicardial coronary arteriolar disease, and congestive heart failure; hemorrhagic and nonhemorrhagic stroke; end-stage renal disease; and dissecting aortic aneurysm and other emergent hypertensive disorders. It is critically necessary to understand the nature of the disease pathophysiologically; by doing so, it is then possible to conceive and to develop new therapies as well as to select pharmacological treatment more rationally. This chapter considers a conception of the pathophysiological alterations associated with the most common form of systemic arterial hypertension, essential hypertension (or primary hypertension).

THE MOSAIC

As already suggested in the Acknowledgments at the beginning of this book, it was approximately 50 years ago when Page described his concept of the mosaic of hypertension. Inherent in his thesis was the belief that hypertension is multifactorial in causation. This is because all of the mechanisms that serve to control arterial pressure in normal patients as well as those with hypertensive disease relate to each other in a kaleidoscopic fashion—each with the others—so that all are critical in maintaining homeostasis, physiologically or pathophysiologically (Figure 1.1). In the case of hypertension, the fundamental driving physiological purpose is to maintain normal tissue perfusion. In hypertension, this is accomplished at the expense of an increased vascular resistance and, hence, the elevated arterial pressure characteristic of hypertensive disease.

Altered Hemodynamics

To understand the pathophysiological alterations associated with the systemic arterial hypertensive diseases, there must first be a clear-cut understanding of the hemodynamic alterations associated with a persistent elevation of arterial pressure. By definition, hypertension is a hemodynamic disorder in which the elevated arterial

Table 1.1. Risk Factors Underlying Coronary Heart Disease

Not treatable
Advancing age
Male gender
Black race
Positive family history

Treatable
Hypertension
Hyperlipidemias
Tobacco consumption
Obesity
Diabetes mellitus

Unresolved (as to whether treatment reverses risk)
Left ventricular hypertrophy
Hyperinsulinism
Hyperuricemia

pressure may be associated with an increased cardiac output or total peripheral resistance (or both). In most patients with essential hypertension, the increased arterial pressure is produced by an increased total peripheral resistance. In some patients, however, an elevated cardiac output may also participate. It is clear that when one considers the magnitude of the elevated arterial pressure, any changes in blood viscosity could not account importantly for such a major pressure increase. Nevertheless, intravascular rheological changes may significantly alter local tissue blood flow dynamics in the major target organs of the disease and, thereby, important organ hemodynamic alterations. Thus, it is very possible that some degree of viscosity increase and changes in rheologic alterations (as will be described below) could serve to exacerbate the altered hemodynamic characteristics of the coronary, renal, and brain circulations. For the most part, however, the increased total peripheral resistance (or, in organ circulations, the vascular resistances) is the hemodynamic hallmark of the hypertensive diseases. Indeed, this increased vascular resistance is more or less uniformly distributed throughout the various organ circulations. The mechanisms responsible for this resistance increase is an augmented vascular smooth muscle tone, primarily in the precapillary arterioles. It provides the explanation for the underlying and fundamental mechanisms accounting for that increased state of the arteriolar contractile state (i.e., arteriolar constriction) that is implicit in the multifactorial nature of the disease (Table 1.2). As already suggested, this textbook will emphasize the mechanisms as they are related to essential hypertension since this primary form of hypertension occurs in approximately 95 percent of all patients with systemic arterial hypertension. However, this pathophysiological discussion will be relevant to certain other (i.e., secondary) clinical forms of hypertension. In doing so, the discussion of the pertinent underlying pressor mechanisms in those secondary forms of hypertension are made for comparison purposes as well as to provide a more comprehensive insight into those that could occur in patients with essential hypertension (Table 1.3).

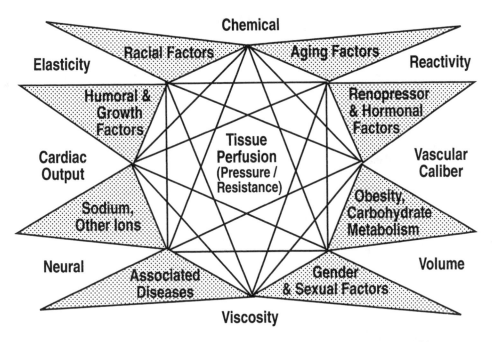

Figure 1.1. The Mosaic of Hypertension. The multifactorial nature of hypertension was proposed originally by I. H. Page and presented in the open areas; additional factors, modified by the author, are presented in the stippled areas. Each of these (and other) factors interrelate with one another in a kaleidoscopic fashion in order to maintain normal tissue perfusion in response to an increasing vascular resistance and at the expense of the abnormally elevated arterial pressure. (Modified from Frohlich ED: Clinical classifications of hypertensive diseases. In: *Atherosclerosis and Coronary Artery Disease* (Fuster V, Ross R, Topol EJ, eds.). Lippincott-Raven, Philadelphia, 1996.)

Arteriolar Constriction As already indicated, the state of arteriolar (and, for that matter, venular) smooth muscle tone is increased in hypertension, although the precise mechanism(s) for this phenomenon is not entirely and precisely known. This, no doubt, relates to the tremendous number of pressor and depressor factors that participate normally in regulating vessel tone and caliber and, hence, arterial pressure. Thus, these factors also participate in the increased vascular resistance in patients with most forms of essential hypertension. Lessons concerning this regulation of increased vascular resistance have been learned from the variety of secondary forms of hypertension in which certain pressor and depressor mechanisms are known to have a major influence in regulating vascular resistance (e.g., angiotensin II in renal arterial disease, catecholamines in pheochromocytoma). Thus, it is very likely that the increased vascular resistance in most patients with essential hypertension is mediated by more than one mechanism. Some of these mechanisms are predetermined by inborn genetic factors since it has become increasingly apparent that much of the pathophysiological alterations in essential hypertension is polygenetic in origin. Furthermore, many of the pressor and depressor mechanisms that seem to be operative have been well documented to actively increase the tone of vascular smooth muscle. Even more exciting (to my way

Table 1.2. Active and Passive Mechanisms of Altering Vascular Resistance

I. Constriction
   A. Active
      1. Adrenergic stimulation (via increased neural input or increased vascular responsiveness to normal neural input)
      2. Catecholamines: norepinephrine, epinephrine, dopamine
      3. Renopressor: angiotensin II
      4. Cations: Ca^{2+}, K^+ (high concentration)
      5. Other humoral substances: vasopressin, serotonin, endothelin, certain prostaglandins
   B. Passive
      1. Edema: extravascular compression
      2. Vessel wall waterlogging
      3. Increased blood or plasma viscosity
      4. Obstruction (proximal): thrombosis, embolus
      5. Hyposmolarity
      6. Temperature: cold (?)
II. Dilation
   A. Active
      1. Acetylcholine
      2. Nitric oxide
      3. Kinins: bradykinin, kallidin
      4. Prostaglandins (certain)
      5. Catecholamines: epinephrine (low dose), dopamine
      6. Histamines
      7. Peptides: atrial natriuretic factor, insulin, secretin, vasoactive intestinal polypeptide, parahormone, calcitonin gene-related peptide, substance P, endorphins, enkephalins
      8. Renal medullary phospholipid substance (medullin)
      9. Cations: K^+ (low concentration), Mg^{2+}
     10. Vasoactive metabolites: adenosine, Krebs intermediate metabolites, acetate
   B. Passive
      1. Reduced blood or plasma viscosity
      2. Increased tonicity
      3. Hyperosmolarity
      4. Temperature: heat

of thinking), many new mechanisms seem to be elucidated with each passing year (Table 1–2). Thus, in the final analysis, vascular smooth muscle tone becomes abnormally increased as a result of one or more of these factors that participate in the underlying disease process. As a consequence of the increased vascular resistance, arterial pressure rises in order to maintain tissue perfusion at the expense of the consequences of the vascular and cardiac damage that secondarily result. These effects are ultimately expressed by altered vessel or cardiac structure as well as by the secondarily induced tissue effects of reduced organ blood flow.

As suggested in Table 1–2, the increased tone of the arteriolar or venular smooth muscle occurs no matter what the mechanism. Thus, whether the myocyte is stimulated by enhanced adrenergic input or elevated circulating levels (or increased vas-

Table 1.3. Classification of the Various Forms of the Systemic Arterial Hypertensions

Primary (essential) hypertension (hypertension of undetermined cause)
Borderline (labile) essential hypertension
Essential hypertension: systolic pressures greater than 140 mmHg and diastolic pressures greater than 89 mmHg
Isolated systolic hypertension: systolic pressures greater than 139 mmHg with diastolic pressures less than 89 mmHg

Secondary hypertensions
Coarctation of the aorta

Central nervous system diseases
Increased spinal fluid pressure
CNS tumors
Diencephalic syndrome

Renal arterial disease (renovascular hypertension)
Nonatherosclerotic (fibrosing) renal arterial disease
Atherosclerotic renal arterial disease
Aneurysm(s) of renal artery
Embolic renal arterial disease
Extravascular compression (of renal artery): tumor, fibrosis
Perinephric hull (Page kidney)

Renal parenchymal diseases
Chronic pyelonephritis
Acute glomerulonephritis
Chronic glomerulonephritis
Polycystic renal disease
Diabetic nephropathy
Others: amyloidosis, ureteral obstruction, etc.

Hormonal diseases
  Thyroid
    Hyperthyroidism
    Hypothyroidism
    Hashimoto's thyroiditis

  Adrenal cortical hypertension
    Cushing's disease or Cushing's syndrome
    Primary hyperaldosteronism
      Adenoma
      Bilateral hyperplasia
    Adrenal enzyme deficiencies
    Adrenal medullary hypertension (i.e., pheochromocytoma)

  Others: Ectopic production of hormones
  Growth hormone excess

Table 1.3. Classification of the Various Forms of the Systemic Arterial Hypertensions— *continued*

Hypercalcemic disease states (e.g., hyperparathyroidism, milk-alkali syndrome, hypervitaminosis D, idiopathic hypercalcemia)

Drugs, Chemicals, and Foods
Excessive alcohol intake
Excessive dietary sodium intake
Exogenously administered adrenal steroids: birth control pills; adrenal steroids for asthma, malignancies; anabolic steroids
Licorice excess (imported—not synthetic)
Cold preparations: phenylpropanolamine; nasal decongestants
Snuff
"Street drugs" (e.g., cocaine)

Complications from specific therapy
  Antidepressant therapy (tricyclic; antidepressants; MAO inhibitors)
  Chronic steroid administration
  Cyclosporine (transplantation and certain diseases immunosuppressive therapy)
  Beta-adrenergic receptor agonists (e.g., for asthma)
  Radiation nephritis, arteritis
  Lithotripsy therapy for renal calculi

cular responsiveness to catecholamines); alterations in circulating or local autocrine/paracrine effects of humoral substance such as catecholamines and serotonin; local or systemic participation of vasoactive peptides (e.g., angiotensin II, vasoactive intestinal polypeptide, endothelin) or ions (e.g., calcium); or by hemodynamic or structural effects of growth factors (e.g., angiotensin II endothelin, insulin-like growth factor, platelet-derived growth factor [PDGF]). An increased vascular smooth muscle tone results. Alternatively, vascular resistance increase may also be produced by reduced amounts of circulating vasodilating agents (e.g., acetylcholine, histamine, adenosine, prostaglandins), local vasoactive peptides (e.g., insulin, calcitonin gene-related peptide), or ions (e.g., potassium, magnesium, Krebs intermediate metabolites) (Table 1–2). Whatever the myocytic stimulus, there is a consequent rise in cytoplasmic free calcium ions from their resting state and a resulting enhanced phosphorylation of myosin light chains. This increased calcium ionic milieu may be achieved either through an inflow of calcium ions through calcium or other (e.g., alpha-adrenergic) receptor activated membrane channels or by a release of calcium ions from intracellular organelles (primarily the sarcoplasmic reticulum), although it may be released from the mitochondria or from binding with protein substrates. The former receptor-operated channels explain the mechanisms of action of the various membrane receptors of naturally occurring humoral substances or of the various antihypertensive agents (e.g., calcium antagonists). The net result of the intracytoplasmic calcium ion release appears to promote the formation of inositol triphosphate (IP3) and diacylglycerol, with IP3 serving as the second messenger mediating the calcium ion release and the resulting mechanical coupling that permits an enhanced state of contractility of vascular smooth muscle.

Still another factor that participates in the increased vascular resistance of hypertension is an increased wall-to-lumen diameter of the arterial and arteriolar wall. This structural alteration of the vessel wall in hypertension serves to amplify the responsiveness of the arteriole to constrictor stimuli, thereby serving to perpetuate and maintain the hypertensive state. Very recent investigations have suggested that the hemodynamic stress of vessel stretch may be an important mechanism responsible for the vessel wall thickening or even in the myocytic hypertrophy of the left ventricle. Indeed, several recent reports have indicated that upon stretch of the ventricular or arteriolar (e.g., renal, coronary) myocyte, one or more of a vast array of "early genes" or proto-oncogenes (e.g., *c-myc, c-fos, c-jun*) and growth factors (e.g., insulin-like growth factor, platelet-derived growth factor, transforming growth factor beta) may participate in initiating DNA-directed myocytic (and perhaps collagen and other) growth. Some of these growth factors are vasoconstrictors in and of themselves (e.g., angiotensin II, norepinephrine, endothelin), and they may even be produced within the arteriolar or ventricular wall itself. What is all the more intriguing, they (e.g., PDGF) may also participate in atherogenesis and, hence, explain the close relationship of two common and comorbid disease processes (i.e., hypertensive vascular disease and atherosclerosis) that progress, then, in tandem.

Pre- and Post-capillary Constriction   For the most part, all patients with hypertension have an increased arterial pressure that is associated with an increased contractile state of vascular smooth muscle in both the arterioles and venules. Additionally, the wall-to-lumen ratio of the arterioles, which is also increased in hypertension, serves to further increase vascular resistance and arterial pressure. The increased tone of the smooth muscle in the arteriolar wall is responsible for the increased total peripheral resistance. As a result of the arteriolar constriction and, consequently, the increased total peripheral resistance and arterial pressure, left ventricular afterload increases *pari passu*. This provides the major hemodynamic determinant for the associated adaptive left ventricular hypertrophy and eventual hypertensive heart disease. These precapillary changes of the entire systemic circulation are also associated with generalized constriction of the postcapillary venules that reduce total body venous capacity. It is these simultaneous constricting effects of arteriolar and venular constriction that relate to several pathophysiological phenomena and consequences of hypertensive disease.

The reduced venous capacity that results from postcapillary venular constriction diminishes the overall venular capacity of the peripheral circulation. As a result, circulating intravascular volume is redistributed from the periphery to the central circulation to increase venous return to the heart and, hence, cardiac output. This intravascular volume redistribution phenomenon has been demonstrated clinically in patients with essential hypertension as well as in several experimental forms of hypertension. Early in the development of hypertension, this systemic venoconstriction may not be associated with intravascular volume contraction. Later, however, as the severity of arteriolar and venular constriction progresses further, capillary hydrostatic pressure increases and circulating intravascular volume diminishes. This is probably the consequence of two factors: (1) movement of plasma from the circulation into the extravascular compartment and (2) excretion of circulating volume by the kidneys as arterial pressure increases (i.e., the phenomenon of pressure natriuresis). Therefore, as hypertensive vascular disease progresses and becomes more severe with more intense arteriolar and venular constriction, intravascular volume progressively contracts, resulting in increased circulating blood (and plasma) viscosity, increased plasma protein concentration, and elevated hemoglobin and hematocrit. This concept of both pre- and postcapillary constriction in hypertension is a useful pathophysiological consideration for a number of practical clinical implications (Figure 1–2).

High Hematocrit and Hemoglobin   First, it explains why there is a "reactive" or "relative" polycythemia that can be detected frequently in patients with essential hypertension. Gaisböck reported about this phenomenon at the turn of the century when he described a polycythemia associated with essential hypertension. Unlike polycythemia *rubra vera,* there is neither a leukocytosis or thrombocytosis nor is there splenomegaly associated with the hypertension. The elevated hemoglobin and hema-

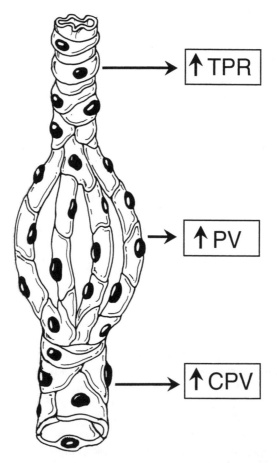

Figure 1.2. This diagram demonstrates the differential roles of precapillary (arteriolar) constriction in increasing total peripheral resistance and postcapillary (venular) constriction in translocating intravascular volume from the periphery to the central circulation. Alternately, severe postcapillary constriction will increase capillary hydrostatic pressure and favor capillary ultrafiltration to extravascular tissue sites.

tocrit (of the Gaisböck syndrome) that is frequently found in the ruddy patient with essential hypertension is associated with a contracted plasma volume. This increase in red cell mass and reduction in plasma volume has actually been measured in a large number of patients with essential hypertension. In these patients, the intravascular (i.e., plasma) volume was found to be contracted in direct relationship to the height of arterial pressure and total peripheral resistance. A similar phenomenon has also been demonstrated in patients with hypertension and renal arterial disease and with pheochromocytoma. In contrast with those findings, in other patients with hypertension (e.g., with renal parenchymal disease, primary aldosteronism, or other steroidal forms of hypertension) and in some patients with more volume-dependent essential hypertension, the magnitude of plasma volume is directly related to the height of arterial pressure. This, then, provides an explanation why those patients with essential hypertension with plasma volume contraction may lose effective control of arterial pressure when they are treated only with an adrenergic inhibitor or a direct smooth muscle relaxing vasodilator. Thus, the plasma volume expands as the pressure is reduced with treatment, and blood pressure control can then be restored with the addition of a diuretic. Indeed, this explains the phenomenon of pseudotolerance observed with greater frequency when these forms of antihypertensive therapy were more commonly used. Another practical clinical application of this important physiological concept is demonstrated (to the converse) by the wisdom of expanding intravascular volume preoperatively by autotransfusion in the patient with a pheochromocytoma in order to prevent intraoperative hypotension and shock upon the sudden excision of the tumor and reduction in circulating catecholamines.

"Edemas" A second clinical example of the applicability of the coincident pre- and postcapillary vasoconstriction may be demonstrated in those patients with severe hypertensive retinopathy. It provides an explanation for the transudation of protein through the capillary bed in patients with accelerated hypertension as well as for the papilledema associated with malignant hypertension. A third example relates to the development of edema when patients use shorter acting or higher doses of long-acting calcium antagonists. This edema is not the consequence of renal-mediated fluid retention but rather of potent drug-induced precapillary arteriolar dilation associated with postcapillary reflex constriction (particularly with prolonged upright posture).

Nephrosclerosis A fourth example, which is becoming more and more appreciated clinically, relates to the increased intraglomerular hydrostatic pressure in patients with hypertensive nephrosclerosis. Thus, both afferent and efferent glomerular arteriolar constriction occur in patients with prolonged systemic arterial hypertension. This favors glomerular capillary pressure elevation, ultrafiltration, increased protein filtered by the glomerulae, and consequent glomerulosclerosis. It is useful to know that with therapeutic reduction of afferent and efferent arteriolar resistance, glomerular hydrostatic pressure also may also diminish in association with a reduction in protein filtered and reversal or inhibited further progression of glomerular sclerosis. This phenomenon has been demonstrated experimentally and, more recently, clinically with the angiotensin converting enzyme (ACE) inhibitors. These findings have provided some degree of further credibility to the concept that angiotensin II participates in the progression of nephrosclerosis in hypertension. It is suggested that inhibition of angiotensin II generation will provide benefit for those patients so affected. However, at least with the converting enzyme inhibitors, it is possible that the increased kinins resulting from ACE inhibition may also participate in the reversal of these renal pathophysiological alterations. Although these effects have not been demonstrated in end-stage renal disease secondary to essential hypertension, they have been shown in patients with early diabetic nephrosclerosis with and without associated hypertension.

"High Cardiac Output"Hypertension   A fifth example of the phenomenon of pre- and postcapillary constriction provides, in part, a pathophysiological explanation for the increased cardiac output and hyperdynamic circulation that is observed during the development of essential hypertension. Thus, early in the elaboration of hypertension (i.e., in those patients with borderline or "labile" hypertension) when blood pressure is elevated only at times but normal at other times, cardiac output is increased. This increased output, as already suggested above, is related to the translocation of the circulating intravascular volume from the periphery to the central circulation as a result of the postcapillary (i.e., venular) constriction. Although the total peripheral resistance at this stage is said to be normal, we have suggested that it is "inappropriately so" since should cardiac output become elevated to the same extent in a normotensive individual, the total peripheral resistance would be slightly diminished. With progression of the hypertensive vascular disease and as the pre- and postcapillary vasoconstriction increase further, the intravascular (i.e, plasma) volume progressively contracts as described above. This contraction in circulating intravascular volume proportionally diminishes the cardiopulmonary volume, decreases right atrial venous return, and, thus, the cardiac output is reduced to a more normal level (than that which was observed earlier in the disease process in the patients with labile or borderline hypertension and even in those with the less severe stages of essential hypertension).

Fluid Volume Partitions

As originally postulated by Starling, local hemodynamic and other pressure alterations are responsible for the movement of water across the major body fluid compartments. These factors include the local capillary hydrostatic and local tissue pressures as well as the protein oncotic pressures intravascularly and extravascularly. (These considerations have already been described above in our discussion of pre- and postcapillary constriction.) In general, total body water is normal in essential hypertension; moreover, it seems to be normally distributed between the extracellular and intracellular fluid compartments in hypertension. However, although there is much epidemiological evidence for a metabolic derangement in the handling of sodium in patients with hypertension, there is little evidence available to support the concept that total body sodium is increased in hypertensive disease or that it is associated with abnormally expanded total body water. Nevertheless, there is good clinical investigative evidence that the extracellular fluid volume seems to be maldistributed in hypertension. Thus, as intravascular (i.e., plasma) volume becomes contracted in patients with essential hypertension (as a result of the alterations in pre- and postcapillary vessel tone described in the foregoing section as well as by increasing renal perfusion pressures), it is associated with a greater degree of interstitial fluid volume. This movement of fluid from the intravascular to the extravascular (including the interstitial fluid) compartments has very specific pathophysiological implications. As indicated above, in the earlier days of antihypertensive therapy, when arterial pressure was reduced by either the direct-acting smooth muscle vasodilators (e.g., hydralazine, minoxidil) or by the antiadrenergic compounds (e.g., reserpine, methyldopa, ganglion-blocking drugs), capillary hydrostatic and renal arterial perfusion pressures diminish. This pressure reduction permits the migration of fluid from the extravascular compartment (i.e., interstitial fluid) intravascularly to expand (or "reconstitute") the circulating blood volume. The net effect was an attenuation in effectiveness of the prescribed antihypertensive agent. However, with the addition of a diuretic (or by increasing the dosage of the diuretic already used), intravascular volume again becomes contracted, thereby restoring antihypertensive effectiveness of the prescribed treatment program. This discussion, therefore, offers the physiological explanation for the phenomenon of "pseudotolerance." This phenomenon is still encountered in the intensive care unit setting in the patient with severely elevated arterial pressure when increasing doses of sodium nitroprusside must be infused to reduce arterial pressure until a so-called "tachyphylaxis" occurs. In reality, this is not true tachyphylaxis to the nitroprusside but the pseudotolerance that has resulted from intravascular volume expansion. Restoration of effective and well-controlled hypotension occurs with the administration of a diuretic. In more recent years, with the introduction of the beta-adrenergic receptor, angiotensin converting enzyme, and calcium channel inhibitory therapies, the induced hypotension is not usually associated with expanded intravascular volume, and "pseudotolerance" has been of less concern unless the patient's problem is compounded by impaired renal function.

As already indicated, most patients with essential hypertension demonstrate an inverse relationship between height of arterial pressure (or total peripheral resistance) and the magnitude of intravascular volume. This inverse relationship between intravascular volume and arterial pressure has also been demonstrated in other forms of hypertension, including hypertensive patients with renal arterial disease and pheochromocytoma. In contrast, other patients with hypertension may demonstrate a direct relationship between the height of arterial pressure and intravascular volume. These patients may have a steroidal dependent form of hypertension (e.g., primary aldosteronism, Cushing's disease) or renal parenchymal disease, or they may include a small number of patients with essential hypertension having a volume-dependent form of the disease (i.e., low plasma renin activity that is suppressed by the intravascular volume expansion). In this respect, this phenomenon of an expanded intravascular volume in direct relationship with the height of arterial pressure may be encountered even in those patients with parenchymal renal disease who may still have normal renal function tests (e.g., serum creatinine and glomerular filtration rate). These considerations also have important clinical and therapeutic considerations. For example, many clinical studies have shown that patients with low plasma renin activity and essential hypertension are particularly responsive to diuretic therapy.

SODIUM METABOLISM

Many major epidemiological studies have demonstrated a high direct correlation between the magnitude of dietary sodium intake and the prevalence of hypertension in many populations. Moreover, other studies have shown that in those societies with daily sodium dietary intakes of less than 60 millimoles, hypertension is practically non-existent and they fail to show a rise in arterial pressure with aging. Furthermore, other epidemiological studies have demonstrated that there may be genetically determined alterations in sodium transport across cell membranes in different population groups of patients with essential hypertension. Notwithstanding this massive volume of epidemiological data that support an important role for the sodium ion in essential hypertension, there is a relative paucity of pathophysiological data to confirm this thesis clinically. The major problem lies in the elusive ability to define just which patients with essential hypertension are sodium sensitive and which are not. At this point, therefore, the subject still remains one of great controversy. Nevertheless, it would be folly to suggest that there is no evidence to relate an abnormality in sodium metabolism or handling at least in some patients with essential hypertension.

HORMONAL ALTERATIONS

Because of the foregoing issue concerning the role of the sodium ion in essential hypertension, many studies have focused upon the role of adrenal corticosteroids in the pathogenesis of at least some individuals with hypertension. For the most part, there have been few patients with essential hypertension who demonstrate an abnormality of steroidal mechanisms underlying the hypertension disease process. In general, aldosterone seems to be synthesized, released, and excreted in proportion to the levels of stimulation of the renin-angiotensin system in patients with essential hypertension, and there does not seem to be any clear-cut derangement in adrenal steroid biosynthesis in such patients. In those patients with abnormal levels of steroidal biosynthesis and release, the derangements are due to specific adrenal diseases (Cushing's syndrome and disease, primary hyperaldosteronism, hydroxylase deficiencies, etc.). Recent studies in many of these forms of secondary hypertension have demonstrated specific genetic enzymatic abnormalities to account for the steroidal defect.

Hormonal alterations have been demonstrated in other patients with hypertension. There is a high prevalence of hypertension in patients with hyperthyroidism and hypothyroidism. The mechanism of the former type of hypertension relates to an association of increased adrenergic activity with the increase in thyroidal function, but there are no specific explanations for the latter form of hypertension. There also is an increased incidence of hypertension among patients with the broad spectrum of hypercalcemic diseases (including hyperparathyroidism). In this respect, recent studies have suggested an abnormality in the parathyroid hormone that may occur in some patients with essential hypertension, although this recent observation still requires further confirmation and study. In any event, the basic mechanism may be explained on the basis of increased ionizable calcium in the vascular smooth muscle cell. Still other hormonal diseases that have been associated with hypertension include acromegaly and gigantism, ectopically produced hormones associated with tumors and, of course, with exogenously administered hormones (e.g., oral contraceptives, androgens) and other chemicals (e.g., nose drops, licorice, snuff and "street drugs"). In this regard, Table 1-3 presents a classification of the various forms of secondary hypertension based upon the mechanisms involved.

NEURAL MECHANISMS

The autonomic nervous system participates importantly in the normal control of arterial pressure and may be altered in patients with essential hypertension. One would normally expect that as arterial pressure increases, heart rate should slow. However, most patients with essential hypertension (no matter what the severity) demonstrate a faster resting heart rate than normal, even if frank tachycardia is not present. This is but one manifestation of the phenomenon of resetting or altered baroreceptor sensitivity in hypertension. In addition, increased release, sensitivity, and excretion of norepinephrine has been repeatedly demonstrated in patients with essential hypertension, more frequently in patients with borderline or with the lesser stages of severity of the disease. These findings have been supported by the demonstration of increased serum catecholamine concentration in general proportion to the altered hemodynamics in these patients. The elevation in catecholamine concentration in those patients with essential hypertension, however, is not nearly as great as that observed in those patients with pheochromocytoma.

It is of interest that in those patients with lesser degrees of severity of essential hypertension, particularly those with a hyperdynamic circulatory state (with or without idiopathic mitral valve prolapse syndrome), serum catecholamine concentration may be increased. This finding may provide an explanation for the altered hemodynamic findings as well as the augmented myocardial contractility, the idiopathic mitral valve prolapse, and the associated cardiac dysrhythmias. In general, there have been no alterations reported in catecholamine biosynthesis or in release of these substances, although reports of increased responsiveness of adrenergic receptor sites have been reported in patients as well as in certain experimental forms of hypertension. Indeed, we have reported that certain patients with essential hypertension with evidence of a hyperdynamic circulation have demonstrated an increased beta-adrenergic receptor responsiveness to isoproterenol infusion, higher than normal levels of norepinephrine, provocation of a hysterical response to low-dose infusion rates of the beta-receptor agonist, occasional idiopathic mitral valvular prolapse, and reversal of these findings with beta-adrenergic blocking agent therapy (*vide infra*). The increased responsiveness of blood vessels to catecholamine stimulation and stressful stimuli (including cold and physiological interventions) has not usually been related to receptor-mediated events, although for many years increased cold pressor stimulation responsiveness had been thought to be characteristic of patients with essential hypertension. Furthermore, we have also reported altered responses to upright tilting, Valsalva maneuvers, and tyramine stimulation of norepinephrine release from nerve endings may provide a useful indication of adrenergic neural participation in certain patients with essential hypertension. Thus, patients with milder forms of hypertension may demonstrate orthostatic hypertension and a greater degree of diastolic pressure overshoot during the Valsalva maneuver, suggesting a greater neural component in patients with orthostatic hypertension. In contrast, those patients at the opposite extreme with a history of more severe hypertension (e.g., malignant hypertension or hypertension associated with congestive heart failure) may demonstrate orthostatic hypotension and a lesser degree of pressure-overshoot immediately following release from the Valsalva maneuver.

Several years ago, a clonidine suppression test was introduced to differentiate those patients with pheochromocytoma from those patients with essential hypertension having slightly elevated levels of plasma catecholamines. Clonidine administration into patients with essential hypertension will suppress elevated catecholamine levels if elevated. In contrast, the elevated catecholamine levels will not suppress to normal in patients with pheochromocytoma. Thus, following administration of the centrally active adrenergic inhibitor clonidine (0.l mg hourly for three doses) the patients with essential hypertension and elevated catecholamine levels will suppress their circulating catecholamine concentration to the normal range. However, those patients with elevated catecholamine levels resulting from pheochromocytoma will not demonstrate that suppression.

RENOPRESSOR SYSTEM

The enzyme renin is released from the juxtaglomerular (J-G) apparatus of the kidney upon stimulation by reduced renal flow and/or perfusion pressure, intravascular volume contraction, decreases in dietary sodium intake, beta-adrenergically mediated neural input to the J-G apparatus, reduced plasma levels of aldosterone, and so on (Table 1.4). This release of the renal enzyme acts on its circulating peptide-protein substrate angiotensinogen which is produced by the liver. The result is the liberation of the decapeptide angiotensin I from its protein substrate which is immediately transformed in the pulmonary circulation by the angiotensin converting enzyme by cleaving off a terminal dipeptide to form the powerful pressor octapeptide angiotensin II. Angiotensin II then acts on its target sites: vascular smooth muscle to produce vasoconstriction; adrenal cortex to release aldosterone; adrenal medulla to release catecholamines; certain medullary centers in the brain to initiate adrenergic outflow from the brain; and thirst centers in the brain that promote fluid intake. The net result is a defense of arterial pressure by increasing vascular resistance and retention of sodium and water. The negative feedback to this homeostatic physiological sequence occurs when, in the presence of excess angiotensin II, renin release is inhibited.

However, angiotensin II may not only be produced by this classical endocrine mechanism. Recently, another alternative means of angiotensin II generation has been demonstrated—in the heart, for example. Thus, another enzyme (i.e., chymase) is also produced in the heart which directly also serves to convert angiotensin I to II without the aid of the angiotensin converting enzyme. Recent studies suggest that this mechanism of angiotensin II production predominates in the human heart. In addition, it is now clear that the entire renin-angiotensin system is produced locally in a number of organ cellular systems in heart, vessel wall, brain, ovary, salivary gland, uterus, and liver. This concept has been controversial until recently because the one point requiring further clarification is whether the enzyme renin is actually produced locally in heart and arterial wall since it may be delivered to these sites through the bloodstream. However, each of the other components of the renin-angiotensin system have been demonstrated to be

Table 1.4. Mechanisms of Increased Renin Release from the Kidney

- Reduced renal blood flow and/or perfusion pressure
- Contracted intravascular volume
- Dietary sodium restriction (<100 mEq/day)
- Increased β-adrenergically mediated neural input
- Reduced aldosterone levels in blood
- Upright posture
- Hormones or humoral agents (e.g., catecholamines)
- Drugs (e.g., diuretics)

produced locally. (More recently, some reports have suggested that the adrenal steroid aldosterone may also be produced locally in the heart.) The precise roles for these local systems are not yet clearly known but much has been written already about the intracellular generation of angiotensin II on muscle protein synthesis with its inherent implications in the development or regression of vascular and ventricular hypertrophy. Local generation of angiotensin II may be of particular importance in (a) the function of the cell (e.g., the cardiac or arteriolar myocyte) which produced the peptide (an *intracrine* function), (b) the effect on neighboring cells (an *autocrine* function or role), or (c) association with other hormones (e.g., kinins, catecholamines, atrial natriuretic peptide, endothelin) within that organ (a *paracrine* function) (Figure 1.3).

Measurement of plasma renin activity (PRA) has important clinical implications not only in the classification of patients with essential hypertension but in other hypertensive diseases. Thus, if an adrenal steroidal form of hypertension is suspected (e.g., primary aldosteronism), PRA will be suppressed; and this will be associated with an expanded plasma volume, hypokalemic alkalosis, and increased urinary (or plasma levels of) aldosterone and, of course, with the anatomical demonstration of the adrenal tumor (by imaging techniques or at surgery). In contrast, if elevated levels of PRA are demonstrated and renal arterial disease is suspected, then collection of blood from both renal veins with an inferior vena cava sample below the level of

Systemic and Local Renin-Angiotensin Systems

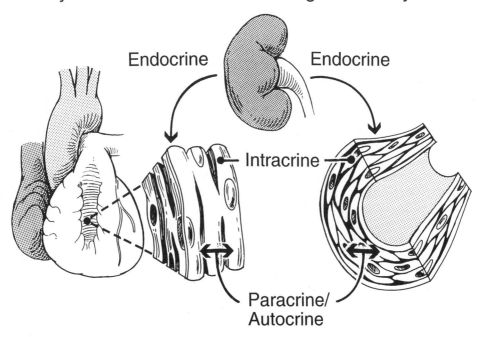

Figure 1.3. This cartoon represents not only the classical endocrine role of the renin-angiotensin system, but also the additional means for the generation of angiotensin II locally within heart, the arteriolar wall, and other organs. See text for further discussion.

the kidneys will be useful in the diagnosis of functionally significant renal arterial disease with hypertension. Lateralization of the tumor will be aided by a PRA ratio of 1.6, with the affected kidney being greater. The diagnosis should be supported by appropriate arteriographic techniques demonstrating the arterial lesion more precisely.

Much interest has been engendered in recent years about the role of the renin-angiotensin system in patients with essential hypertension. Laragh and his colleagues have suggested that patients with essential hypertension may be classified (or "profiled") according to the levels of PRA which must also be expressed with respect to 24-hour sodium excretion. (It must be recognized that PRA will be increased in those patients with reduced dietary sodium intake (less than 100 mEq sodium); and, conversely, PRA will be reduced in those patients with excessive dietary sodium intake.) This categorization has been used not only conceptually with respect to the pathophysiological alterations of the disease but also for selecting antihypertensive therapy on a physiological basis. In general, the levels of PRA are directly related to the generated angiotensin II and to the production and release and excretion of the adrenal cortical hormone aldosterone. These investigators have also suggested that the level of PRA may provide useful prognostic markers. Thus, those patients with high PRA may be at increased risk of premature cardiovascular, stroke, and other morbid and mortal events, whereas those with low PRA may be of lesser risk. Indeed, in one recent report, they suggested that those patients with high PRA were more likely to develop myocardial infarction. Although no precise physiological mechanism was offered to explain this association, employing the foregoing physiological concepts described above, it is possible to suggest one. We do know that the higher the arterial pressure and the more severe the disease, the greater will be the total peripheral resistance; consequently, a more contracted intravascular volume will result. Furthermore, the more contracted the intravascular volume, the greater will be the PRA. With contraction of intravascular volume, blood and plasma viscosity would also increase; and this would be expressed on a microcirculatory level in the coronary or cerebral circulation by augmented protein concentration (including fibrinogen levels) and, hence, greater predisposition for thromboses. Furthermore, even more recent work has suggested that angiotensin II could inhibit an endogenously produced thrombolytic inhibitory factor in blood. These changes may therefore predispose a more viscous coronary microcirculation to a greater likelihood of clot formation. Clearly, the subject remains of great clinical interest, demanding further clarification.

It is particularly pertinent at this point to consider again that hormones, vasoactive substances, and other chemicals and growth factors not only act at their own "classical" target organs, but also may modify the actions of other blood, neurally borne, or local substances. In this fashion, certain agents may exert their physiological actions most subtly by acting in concert with other substance . It is well known, for example, that angiotensin II can augment or amplify adren rgic function by its interaction in certain brain centers as well as at peripheral ganglionic or postganglionic areas by interacting with norepinephrine. Angiotensin may also interact with kinins and prostaglandins in kidney; atrial peptides at nerve endings or at the vascular smooth muscle membrane; and other peptides (e.g., endothelin, neuropeptide Y or substance P) at the vascular smooth muscle membrane or intracellularly. Another possible example of this modulatory cardiovascular action occurs at the endothelial level (with L-arginine, nitric oxide, bradykinin, etc.) to alter local hemodynamic functions. We are now aware that endothelial dysfunction of the foregoing factors occurs in hypertension, atherosclerosis, aging, patients with a history of cigarette smoking, hyper-lipidemias, and in post-menopausal women without estrogen replacement therapy.

We anticipate that within the next few years there will be a tremendous amount of fundamental information that will be generated. We already know that nitric oxide, locally produced in the endothelium of vascular smooth muscle and in the heart (in the coronary arteries as well as the ventricle), is responsible for normal vasodilation and cardiac function. Abnormal nitric oxide synthesis in the endothelium has already been shown to occur in the forearm and coronary circulations in patients with hypertension and experimentally in the glomerulus and renal arteriolae in experimental forms of hypertensi.

ANNOTATED BIBLIOGRAPHY

Freis ED: Hemodynamics of hypertension. *Physiol Rev* 1960;40:27–54.
    A remarkable and classical paper that provides a basis for the hemodynamic derangements of hypertensive vascular disease.
Guyton AC, Granger HJ, Coleman TG: Autoregulation of the total systemic circulation and its relation to control of cardiac output and arterial pressure. *Circ Res* 1971;28(Suppl I):93–97.
    A classical presentation of the systems analysis postulating the role of the kidney in the pathogenesis of hypertension through the phenomenon of total body autoregulation.*
Folköw B: The Fourth Volhard Lecture. Cardiovascular structural adaptation: Its role in the initiation and maintenance of primary hypertension. *Clin Sci Mol Med* 1978;55:3–225.
    An exposition of the structural derangements of the artery and arteriole (increased wall-to-lumen diameter) in hypertension.
Linzbach AJ: Heart failure from the point of view of quantitative anatomy. *Am J Cardiol* 1960;5:370–382.
    A description of the anatomical adaptation of the ventricle to pressure and volume overload.
Meerson FZ: Compensatory hyperfunction, hyperadaptation, and insufficiency of the heart. In: *The Failing Heart: Adaptation and Deadaptation* (Katz AM, ed). Raven Press, New York, 1983, pp. 47–66.
    A special supplement from this Russian pathophysiologist on the functional and structural adaptations of the ventricle to pressure overload.
Grossman W: Cardiac Hypertrophy: Useful adaptation or pathologic process? *Am J Med,* 1980;69:576–584.
    An excellent discussion on the functional adaptation of the ventricle to pressure overload.
Kumuro I, Sibazaki Y, Kurabayashi M, Takaku F, Yazaki Y: Molecular cloning of gene sequences from rat heart rapidly responsive to pressure overload. *Circ Res* 1990;66:979–985.

---

*The concept for the central role of the kidney in the pathophysiology of hypertension and in the phenomenon of pressure-natriuresis.

The first report demonstrating that the initial functional derangement of the ventricle (myocytic stretch) initiates the process of hypertrophy through stimulating DNA mediated protein synthesis. A model for many subsequent studies.

Ross RC, Bowen-Pope DP, Raines EW: Platelets, macrophages, endothelium, and growth factors. Their effects upon cells and their possible roles in atherogenesis. In: *Atherosclerosis* (KT Lee, ed). *Annals NY Acad Sci* 1985;454:254–260.

Libby P, Warner SJC, Salomon RN, Birinyi LK: Production of platelet-derived growth factor-like mitogen by smooth-muscle cells from human atheroma. *N Engl J Med* 1988;318:1493–1498.

Sarzani R, Arnaldi G, Takasaki I, Brecher P, Chobanian AV: Effects of hypertension and aging on platelet-derived growth factor and platelet-derived growth factor receptor expression in rat aorta and heart. *Hypertension* 1991,18(Suppl III): 93–99.

The above two references provide excellent discussions on how local vascular growth factors participate in atherogenesis. Most interestingly, these mitogenic factors in atherosclerosis may be the same factors that participate in hypertension, thereby offering a conceptual explanation as to how one disease exacerbates the other. Sarzani provides such supporting evidence.

Page IH: *Hypertension Mechanisms.* Orlando, FL: Grune and Stratton, 1987.

Page IH: Pathogenesis of arterial hypertension. *JAMA* 1949;140:451–458.

Frohlich ED: (State of the Art): The first Irvine H. Page lecture: The mosaic of hypertension: past, present, and future. *J Hypertension* 1988;6(Suppl 4):S2–S11.

Frohlich ED, Apstein C, Chobanian AV, Devereux RB, Dustan HP, Dzau V, Fauad-Tarazi F, Horan MJ, Marcus M, Massie B, Pfeffer MA, Ré RN, Roccella EJ, Savage D, Shub C: The heart in hypertension. *N Engl J Med* 1992;327:998–1008.

The foregoing reference is a recent summary of the heart in hypertension by working group of the National Heart, Lung, and Blood Institute. Three preceeding references provide discussions on the mosaic concept of Page relating the multifactorial nature of hypertension and left ventricular hypertrophy.

Frohlich ED, Kozul VJ, Tarazi RC, Dustan HP: Physiological comparison of labile and essential hypertension. *Circ Res* 1970;27(1):55–69.

Frohlich ED, Tarazi RC, Dustan HP: Clinical–physiological correlations in the development of hypertensive heart disease. *Circulation* 1971;44:446–455.

Dunn FG, Chandraratna P, de Carvalho JGR, Basta LL, Frohlich ED: Pathophysiologic assessment of hypertensive heart disease with echocardiography. *Am J Cardiol* 1977;39:789–795.

The above three references are clinical pathophysiological studies describing the development of labile and essential hypertension. The latter reference provides that first support to the former discussions on the clinical, structural, and functional progression of hypertensive heart disease.

Tarazi RC, Dustan HP, Frohlich ED, Gifford RW Jr, Hoffman GC: Plasma volume and chronic hypertension. Relationship to arterial pressure levels in different hypertensive diseases. *Arch Intern Med* 1970;125:835–842.

Tarazi RC: Hemodynamic role of extracellular fluid volume. *Circ Res* 1976; 38(Suppl II):73–83.

Dustan HP, Tarazi RC, Frohlich ED: Functional correlates of plasma renin activity in hypertensive patients. *Circulation* 1970;41:555–567.

These three references are studies that develop the concept of fluid volume alterations in the clinical hypertensions. The functional correlates of PRA in patients with essential hypertension.

Sealey JE, Laragh JH: The renin-angiotensin-aldosterone system for normal regulation of blood pressure and sodium and potassium homeostasis. In: *Hypertension: Pathophysiology, Diagnosis and Management.* (Laragh JH and Brenner BM, eds). Raven Press, New York, 1990, pp. 1287–1317.

Bühler FR, Laragh JH, Baer L, Vaughan ED Jr, Brunner HR: Propranolol inhibition of renin secretion: A specific approach to diagnosis and treatment of renin-dependent hypertensive diseases. *N Engl J Med* 1972;287:1209–1214.

Alderman MH, Madhavan S, Ooi WL, Cohan H, Sealey JE, Laragh JH: Association of the renin sodium profile with the risk of myocardial infarction in patients with hypertension. *N Engl J Med* 1991;324:1098–1104.

The first two references provide the concept and therapeutic rationale for the profiling of PRA in hypertension, the second and third references relate to the profiling to hypertensive outcomes.

Chapter 2

Evaluation of the Patient

As with all clinical problems, it is essential to evaluate the patient thoroughly before one considers management and treatment. This is particularly pertinent in the patient with systemic arterial hypertension for, if therapy is initiated before one completes the overall clinical evaluation, important clues may be distorted. Consider, for example, the patient who is currently taking as simple and straight forward treatment as a thiazide diuretic. The metabolic changes that could be associated with this form of therapy may distort the general clinical status of the patient, including presence of other cardiovascular risk factors. Thus, is the diuretic maybe responsible for the: hypokalemia; slightly elevated serum creatinine concentration; hyperuricemia; or the blood glucose, lipid, and calcium levels? This chapter considers the important clues that may be obtained from a meaningful personal and family history of the patient, the physical examination, and the basic laboratory studies.

FAMILY HISTORY

As indicated at the outset of this book, hypertension is a multifactorial disease. One striking feature of this concept is the very strong family history of hypertension. Indeed, when there is such a history, there is less possibility of the secondary causes for hypertension. However, even when this occurs, one should consider a secondary form of hypertension if the patient has had a long-standing history of well-controlled hypertension, a recent history of sudden onset of hypertension in a child or older person or refractoriness to an effective antihypertensive therapy. Thus, in the patient with a family history of hypertension or of premature cardiovascular death (e.g., from myocardial infarction, "heart failure," "heart attacks," stroke, kidney failure), there is less likelihood of secondary forms of hypertension. Moreover, should any of the secondary forms of hypertension be established, it is also possible that the patient has essential hypertension additionally. After all, essential hypertension is present in about 20 percent of the overall population.

On the other hand, particularly in patients with a family history of premature death, it is important to search for other important cardiovascular risk factors including obesity, diabetes mellitus (any expression of carbohydrate intolerance), elevated blood lipids (including cholesterol and triglycerides), and smoking. Most importantly, should this occur in both parents there are two important considerations: first, there is the obvious assumption that since hypertension is a polygenetic disease, there is a greater likelihood that the pressor mechanisms that are involved are greater and that the disease is, perhaps, more complex; and, secondly, there is greater likelihood that the hypertensive disease is more severe in these patients. Finally, the recent recommendations advanced in JNC-VI take into consideration coexistent cardiovascular risk factors as well as comorbid conditions in selecting antihypertensive treatment and management.

CLINICAL HISTORY

In most patients with systemic hypertension generally there are no other clinical manifestations than the elevated systolic and/or diastolic pressures. Therefore, unless blood pressure is measured in all patients, hypertension will remain unrecognized and, most importantly, untreated. Unless this consideration is kept in mind there will be no further improvement in the control rates of hypertensive disease. Indeed, the data published in JNC-VI indicates that we are already losing ground in that battle.

It has been said that the most common symptoms related to hypertension are fatigue, headache, and epistaxis. These symptoms, however, are among the more common complaints offered by any patient seeking medical attention. Thus, when symptoms are present, they are more likely to be related to the "target organ" involvement (i.e., heart, kidneys, brain) from hypertensive cardiovascular disease. In this regard, the more common complaints include diminished exercise tolerance, easy fatiguability, nocturia, and sensory or motor deficit as evidence for cardiac, renal, and neural involvement, respectively. It is important to question more specifically for the more subtle signs so that, in those patients having earlier stages of hypertension, there may be symptoms of cardiac awareness (e.g., palpitations, a feeling of "skipped heart beats," and tachycardia that may persist inordinately long after exertion or stress). Some patients may complain of heat intolerance or skin flushing of the face and upper chest. These latter signs occur frequently in younger men and women with essential hypertension and, when they are most pronounced, frequently suggest the possibility of thyrotoxicosis, pheochromocytoma, carcinoid syndrome, or the existence of the hyperdynamic beta-adrenergic circulatory state. The chances of these diagnoses being confirmed are highly unlikely; but I usually say to physicians raising these points, that if these diagnoses come to mind, it certainly is worth following through. If we don't pursue such leads in these patients, such diagnoses will never be made. Of course, the classic appearance of the middle-aged man with a florid complexion as being the ideal patient with essential hypertension is highly consistent with Gaisböck's syndrome, which includes hypertension, high hemoglobin and hematocrit, and "relative" or "stress" polycythemia (i.e., contracted plasma volume with normal red cell mass). Chest pain may occur in patients with cardiac involvement even in the absence of occlusive atherosclerotic epicardial coronary arterial disease. The chest pain results from the consequence of the increased myocardial oxygen demand associated with high pressure and left ventricular hypertrophy. Easy fatigability should suggest reduced myocardial function and/or coexisting coronary artery disease.

The most common symptom of early renal involvement in hypertension is nocturia resulting from the diminished renal concentrating ability associated with nephrosclerosis. Hematuria should suggest a secondary form of hypertension, such as renal arterial disease or glomerulonephritis, although this may more likely be related to prostatic hyperplasia or prostate infection in men and urinary tract infection in women. Other causes of hematuria, of course, should include renal cysts, renal stones, and urinary tract neoplasia. Symptoms and signs of neurological deficit (even if transitory) should suggest transient ischemic attacks, lacunar infarcts, or more obvious strokes (due to hemorrhage or thrombosis). When these symptoms occur in patients with atrial fibrillation, always consider the possibility of embolism.

PHYSICAL EXAMINATION

There is no interaction on physical examination on which the diagnosis of hypertension is more dependent than the precise measurement of blood pressure.

Blood Pressure Measurement

As indicated repeatedly, hypertension can neither be controlled nor can its complications be prevented if blood pressure measurement is not routinely and properly obtained on every physical examination. This should be done by all primary care physicians, specialists, dentists and other health care professionals. However, it is important to emphasize that the diagnosis of hypertension should not be made on the basis of any single measurement. Repeated measurements should be obtained during each individual examination, and the diagnosis is established if these blood pressure measurements are elevated on three successive office visits (including the first examination). The American Heart Association and the Joint National Committee have recommended follow-up procedures for repeated measurements based upon the initial measurements (Table 2.1).

These recommendations advise the use of a systematic technique including the purpose and meaning of the blood pressure measurements with advice as to follow-up determinations. Further, should the patient assist in follow-up with home blood pressure measurements, the instrument should be calibrated and validated periodically (once annually). (see Table 2.1)

Ophthalmoscopy The small vessels of the optic fundus provide an excellent means for assessing the degree of systemic vasoconstriction; this examination should be

---

TABLE 2.1. Procedure for Indirect Measurement of Blood Pressure.

- Patients should be seated with their arm bared, supported, and at heart level. They should not have smoked or ingested caffeine within 30 minutes before measurement.
- Measurement should begin after at least five minutes of rest.
- The appropriate cuff size must be used to ensure an accurate measurement. The bladder should nearly (at least 80%) or completely encircle the arm.
- Measurements should be taken with a mercury sphygmomanometer, a recently calibrated aneroid manometer, or a calibrated electronic device.
- Both the systolic and diastolic pressure should be recorded. Disappearance of sound (phase V) should be used for the diastolic reading.
- Two or more readings separated by 2 minutes should be averaged. If the first two readings differ by more than 5 mmHg, additional readings should be obtained.

In addition, I recommend:

- blood pressure should be measured in both arms on the initial physical examination and periodically thereafter. It is not unusual that the measured pressure will be reduced after several years in those elderly patients with occlusive brachial arterial disease at a later date after the initial examination.

performed routinely. The earliest stage (Group I) of hypertensive vascular disease is recognized by increased arterial tortuosity and mild constriction. Coexisting arteriosclerotic changes are manifested by the discontinuity of the arterioles at arteriovenous (AV) crossings (i.e., AV nicking; Group II). Appearance of exudates and hemorrhages (Group III) signals accelerated hypertension; and with the appearance of papilledema (Group IV) malignant hypertension is established. The American Ophthalmological Association has offered a more detailed classification that is based upon the degree of narrowing of both the retinal arterioles and venules (Table 2.2).

Peripheral Pulses

One should always compare the femoral and brachial arterial pulsations in all patients with hypertension in order to search for any delay in the propagation of the aortic pulse wave which should suggest the presence of aortic coarctation (particularly in younger patients). Whereas this diagnosis should be considered in adult patients although it may also provide evidence of atherosclerotic occlusive processes in older patients. In that regard, asymmetrical pressures taken at the brachial arteries should also suggest atherosclerotic occlusive arterial disease. Moreover, this diagnosis should always be considered when (on succeeding patient visits) there is a dramatic or unexplained reduction in arterial pressure in pressures taken in one arm. Clearly, if that occurs, it is wise to measure pressure in the contralateral arm. Auscultation of the carotid arteries for systolic bruits may provide

Table 2.2. Classification of Hypertensive Retinopathy.

A. Keith-Wagener-Barker Classification
    Group I—tortuosity, minimal constriction
    Group II—above + arteriovenous nicking
    Group III—above + hemorrhages and exudates
    Group IV—papilledema
B. American Ophthalmological Society Committee Classification (Wagener-Clay-Gipner)
    1. Generalized arteriolar constriction
        Grade 1—arterioles 3/4 of normal caliber; A/V ratio of 1:2
        Grade 2—arterioles 1/2 of normal caliber; A/V ratio of 1:3
        Grade 3—arterioles 1/3 of normal caliber; A/V ratio of 1:4
        Grade 4—arterioles thread-like or invisible
    2. Focal arteriolar constriction or sclerosis
        Grade 1—localized arteriolar narrowing to 2/3 caliber of proximal segment
        Grade 2—localized arteriolar narrowing to 1/2 caliber of proximal segment
        Grade 3—localized arteriolar narrowing to 1/3 caliber of proximal segment
        Grade 4—arterioles invisible beyond focal constriction
    3. Generalized sclerosis
        Grade 1—increased light-striping; mild AV nicking
        Grade 2—coppery arteriolar color; moderate AV nicking; veins almost completely
                invisible below arteriolar crossing
        Grade 3—silver arteriolar color; severe AV nicking
        Grade 4—arterioles visible only as fibrous cords without bloodstreams
    4. Hemorrhage and exudates—grades 1 to 4 (based on number of affected quadrants
        divided by 2)
    5. Papilledema—grades 1 to 4 (based on diopters of elevation)

signs of preventable strokes and transient ischemic attacks (especially if associated with neurological signs and symptoms); and funduscopy may reveal cholesterol emboli in the retinal arterioles. In this regard, it is important to dissociate bruits heart over the carotid arteries from transmission of aortic systolic ejection-type murmurs. This usually can be clarified by listening carefully for the timing and character of the bruits. Renal arterial bruits on examination of the abdomen, flanks, and back provide an important sign of renovascular hypertension. Systolic bruits are commonly detected, especially in older patients, and may not be associated with occlusive arterial disease. However, when the abdominal bruit is associated with a diastolic component of that bruit, renal arterial disease becomes much more likely and should be carefully and energetically pursued.

Cardiac Examination

Even before cardiac structure is altered (particularly in young, male patients), palpation of the precordium may reveal a hyperdynamic apical impulse and a faster heart rate as evidence of functional hyperdynamic cardiac changes. But, as the heart adapts structurally to the increasing afterload by development of left ventricular hypertrophy, the increased left ventricular mass may not be detectable by the chest roentgenogram or electrocardiogram; echocardiographic assessment is more sensitive. Nevertheless, the earliest clinical index of cardiac involvement in hypertension is left atrial enlargement, which may be suspected by an atrial diastolic gallop (fourth heart sound or the "bruit de gallop"). This finding is highly concordant with at least two of four electrocardiographic criteria of left atrial abnormality (Table 2.3). As detailed below, hemodynamic and echocardiographic studies have demonstrated that when electrocardiographic evidence of left atrial abnormality is demonstrable (even without other clinical indication of left ventricular hypertrophy), there is adequate evidence of impaired left ventricular systolic function. And, as left ventricular hypertrophy becomes more evident, there is palpable evidence of its occurrence by the presence of a sustained left ventricular lift (or "heave") and further impairment of contractile function. Eventually, in patients with severe left ventricular hypertrophy, the presence of a third heart sound (ventricular diastolic gallop) connotes the presence of early left ventricular failure. In those patients with a very high arterial pressure, an aortic diastolic murmur may

---

Table 2.3. Abnormal Diagnostic Electrocardiographic Criteria.

1. Left atrial abnormality (ECG)—two of four of the following criteria
   a. P wave in Lead II ≥ 0.3 mv and ≥ 0.12 sec
   b. Bipeak interval in notched P wave ≥ 0.04 sec
   c. Ratio of P wave duration to PR segment ≥ 1.6 (lead II)
   d. Terminal atrial forces (in V_1)≥ 0.04 sec
2. Left ventricular hypertrophy
   a. Ungerleider index $\geq +15\%$ (chest x-ray alone)
   b. Ungerleider index $\geq +10\%$ (chest x-ray + two of the following ECG criteria)
      (1) Sum of tallest R and deepest S waves ≥ 4.5 mv (precordial)
      (2) LV "strain"—i.e., QRS and T wave vectors 180° apart
      (3) QRS frontal axis $<0°$
   c. All three ECG criteria (above)

occur as the result of a functional eversion of the aortic cusp by the elevated pressure and total peripheral resistance. The more frequently heard precordial or vascular systolic ejection murmur suggests either outflow tract obstruction from aortic stenosis (associated with aging) or a hemic murmur related to a hyperkinetic circulation.

Other Physical Findings

The so-called "buffalo hump," seen on the back below the neck, suggests the presence of Cushing's syndrome; and this may also be associated with abdominal striae and girdle obesity. Neurofibromatosis should suggest the possible coexistence of pheochromocytoma; and so should *café au lait* spots on the skin. In the days prior to effective antihypertensive therapy, cutaneous ulcerations were seen as manifestations of severely impaired cutaneous blood flow. Appearance of anemia on physical examination in the black patient should suggest coexistent hemoglobinemia; but, perhaps equally important (if not as common), the physician should consider the coexistence of anemia secondary to chronic renal disease (even early stages of impaired renal function). Abdominal examination should be careful not only for the auscultation of bruits (as described above), but also for the presence of the palpable kidneys of polycystic renal disease. When the latter occurs, hepatic cysts should also be sought for as well as secondary polycythemia and, eventually, the presence of aneurysms of the circle of Willis should the clinical situation suggest this possibility.

LABORATORY STUDIES

It is important to discuss with the patient appropriate preparation for laboratory tests. As already suggested, it is wise for these studies to be obtained with the patient off all medications, preferably for at least three to four weeks (Table 2.4). Even a sodium-restricted diet may stimulate adrenal cortical production of aldosterone in sufficient quantities to suggest a state of hyperaldosteronism. Dietary sodium intake in excess of 100 mEq/day (2.3 g) will obviate this possibility. This degree of daily sodium intake may still be effective in either reducing pressure in some patients with hypertension or in enhancing the effectiveness of antihypertensive therapy. On the other hand, it is important to realize that diuretics, laxatives, and even intercurrent gastrointestinal infections (associated with nausea, vomiting, and diarrhea) may produce sufficient volume depletion and electrolyte loss so as to produce a state of secondary hyperaldosteronism and associated hypokalemia and alkalosis. Antihypertensive drugs may have effects lasting for as long as four weeks, thereby providing a false concept of the "baseline" untreated pressure levels. Thus, the thiazide diuretics may have persistent effects for two weeks (or longer) following their discontinuation. Other agents may have even longer effects after they are stopped.

Oral contraceptives may elevate arterial pressure and alter intravascular volume, hemodynamics, and plasma renin activity. A number of commonly used medications that can elevate arterial pressure include sympathomimetic nose drops, nonsteroidal anti-inflammatory compounds, monoamine oxidase inhibitors, and tricyclic antidepressant drugs, cyclosporine, and excessive dietary sodium intake. Always keep in mind that certain "street drugs" (e.g., heroin, cocaine) will elevate blood pressure. For this reason, it is important to obtain an accurate history as to **all** medications that the patient is taking. (A more detailed coverage of complicating therapy is included in the suggested references for this chapter.)

The following discussion is offered to provide a comprehensive interpretation of the results of the commonly used laboratory studies ordered in the evaluation of a patient with hypertension. Certainly, not all of these studies that are discussed below may be necessary in the routine evaluation in any one patient; however, this discussion permits a means for the overall evaluation of the patient with hypertension. Nevertheless, the minimal evaluation should include the complete blood count (without differential); determination of serum creatinine (or blood urea mitogen), potassium, blood sugar, uric acid, and cholesterol (with high- and low-density lipoprotein cholesterol fractions) concentrations, and an electrocardiogram. The fewer the laboratory studies the more cost-effective will be the evaluation; however, modern automated laboratory testing techniques provide more measurements and a more comprehensive evaluation, frequently at no greater cost.

Table 2.4. Laboratory Studies That May Be of Value in the Evaluation of the Patient with Hypertension (See Text for Clinical Justifications).

Complete Blood Count
White blood cell count (and differential)
Hemoglobin concentration
Hematocrit
Adequacy of platelets

Blood Chemistries
Sugar (fasting—2-hour postprandial, or glucose tolerance test, if indicated)
Uric acid concentration
Cholesterol (total and with high- and low-density lipoprotein fractions) and triglyceride concentrations
Renal function (serum creatinine and/or blood urea concentrations)
Serum electrolyte (Na, K, Cl, CO_2) concentrations
Calcium and phosphate concentrations
Total protein and albumin concentration
Hepatic function (alkaline phosphatase, bilirubin, serum glutamic oxaloacetic transaminase, serum glutamic pyruvic transaminase, lactic acid dehydrogenase)
Glycosylated hemoglobin
Thyroid stimulating hormone

Urine Studies
Urinalysis
Microalbuminuria
Urine culture (if history of repeated urinary tract infections)
24-hour collection (protein, Na, K, creatinine)

Cardiac Examinations
Electrocardiogram—standard 12 lead
Limited echocardiogram

Complete Blood Count (CBC)

In addition to assessing the hematologic status of a new patient, the CBC has broader significance. Thus, if anemia is present, the physician should determine whether it is a complication of the disease (e.g., renal parenchymal disease), the side effect of antihypertensive drug therapy (e.g., methyldopa-induced hemolysis), or whether it is related to an associated clinical problem (e.g., hemoglobinopathy). On the other hand, an elevated hemoglobin concentration or hematocrit frequently occurs in patients with essential hypertension. As originally described by Gaisböck, an elevated arterial pressure and "polycythemia" without splenomegaly, leukocytosis or thrombocytosis may be explained physiologically in terms of relative polycythemia since red cell mass and erythropoietin levels are normal. This "polycythemia" of hypertension can be explained on the basis of a contracted plasma volume (as described in the chapter on pathophysiology).

It is also of further value to know the white blood cell count since leukopenia may be a complication of angiotensin-converting enzyme therapy. Thus, a baseline determination may be of value in the course of future care.

Blood Chemistries

Several laboratory tests may be of particular value in evaluating the patient with hypertension (see Table 2.4). The fasting blood glucose concentration may be abnormal since diabetes mellitus is a common comorbid disease with hypertension. Moreover, hypertension, carbohydrate intolerance, insulin insensitivity and hyperlipidemia frequently coexist to increase overall cardiovascular risk. Alternatively, the fasting blood glucose concentration may be normal but, if a two or four hour blood glucose measurement is obtained, it may be elevated, alerting the clinician for other manifestations of diabetes. Indeed, abnormal carbohydrate tolerance has been reported to exist in upwards of 65 percent of patients with essential hypertension; and, as indicated above, it not infrequently coexists with hyperinsulemia. Both of these factors have been shown to confer independent risk for increased cardiovascular morbidity and mortality. The mechanism for this increased risk is not perfectly clear at this time, although it continues to remain a subject of intense study. One favored point of current speculation is that insulin hypersensitivity may be related to impaired end-organ response. Thus, further elevation of insulin levels is necessary, which, in turn, may be related to augmented sympathetic responsiveness. This may be particularly so if the patient is obese. Carbohydrate intolerance may be abetted by diuretics; but in most experts' experience, overt diabetes mellitus does not seem to develop *de novo* in the patient with hypertension taking a diuretic. Thus, some expression of abnormal carbohydrate metabolism frequently precedes the initiation of diuretic therapy. As emphasized, for the first time, in JNC-VI the determination of hemoglobin A_{1c} (HbA_{1c}) is extremely valuable in assessing the potential for the patient's risk for developing complications. This is of particular importance in the patient with hypertension since this patient is at greater risk for the development of left ventricular hypertrophy, end-stage renal disease, and retinopathy. The lower the HbA_{1c} value, the lesser is the risk for these complications from the glycosylation of body proteins. In general, authorities recommend its determination at least annually (and more frequently if the patient's blood sugar concentrations are not in good control).

The serum uric acid determination should also suggest which patients may develop more severe hyperuricemia or even clinical gout with diuretic therapy. Hyperuricemia is an extremely common finding even in untreated patients with essential hypertension. Elevated uric acid concentration has also been shown to be an independent cardiovascular risk factor. Furthermore, in a series of studies from our laboratory, we demonstrated that the higher the serum uric acid concentration in patients with otherwise uncomplicated essential hypertension, the lower will be the renal blood flow and the higher the renal vascular resistance. This rise in serum uric acid concentration, therefore, may reflect early renal hemodynamic functional involvement in hypertension. Moreover, our studies have also shown that the hyperuricemia and renal hemodynamic alterations seem to follow the earliest echocardiographic changes of left ventricular hypertrophy. These findings suggest that early cardiac involvement in hypertension usually precedes evidence of renal hemodynamic involvement in patients with essential hypertension; and when it occurs in the untreated patient, renal hemodynamic involvement is more likely.

It is most important to screen patients with hypertension for hyperlipidemia. The serum total cholesterol determination (with high- and low-density lipoprotein cholesterol concentrations), together with measurement of triglyceride concentration, is of major value for detecting remediable hyperlipidemia and reducing yet another risk factor underlying premature coronary heart disease. Moreover, if there is evidence of hyperlipidemia (particularly elevation of the LDL cholesterol and/or reduction of the HDL cholesterol level) and there is any concern on the part of the physician about exacerbating that preexisting abnormality with antihypertensive therapy, prior lipid screening may permit wiser selection of alternative agents.

The kidney, of course, is a prime target organ of hypertension, and renal functional impairment is a major complication of the disease. Therefore, it is important to determine the serum creatinine (preferable) and/or blood urea nitrogen concentrations in all patients. I usually obtain both tests, and by using the serum creatinine concentration along with urinary creatinine excretion (and the timed—usually 24-hour—urinary volume), it is possible to calculate the creatinine clearance (glomerular filtration rate). Since end-stage renal disease continues to increase in this country and elsewhere it is of vital importance to detect those patients with this potential early, since specific antihypertensive therapy may delay, if not prevent, its development (see Chapter 8). Those patients who are at particular risk are black, have hypertension (with proteinuria or microalbuminuria), or have diabetes mellitus.

Measurement of serum electrolyte concentrations, particularly that of serum **potassium,** is of value in excluding diagnostic possibilities of certain secondary forms of hypertension, including those from steroidal hormone excess as well as those with secondary hyperaldosteronism and the adverse effects of diuretic therapy. In these diseases, the hypokalemia is associated with alkalosis. Many factors may produce hypokalemia (Table 2.5), and very few factors (other than laboratory error or red cell hemolysis) are responsible for hyperkalemia. Determination of serum calcium concentration will exclude hypercalcemia, an alteration that is frequently associated with an increased incidence of hypertension. It is also important to be aware that correction of the hypercalcemia may reduce the abnormally elevated pressure to normotensive levels. Serum magnesium concentration is not a test to order routinely; however, in patients with left ventricular enlargement or cardiac failure with hypokalemia, consider the presence of additional hypomagnesemia.

Table 2.5. Factors Responsible for Hypokalemia.

Dietary Sodium Excess Associated with Diuretic Therapy
Chronic Gastrointestinal Potassium Losses
    Vomiting
    Diarrhea
    Laxative abuse
    Pyloric obstruction
    Nasogastric suction
    Villous adenoma
    Malabsorption syndrome
    Ureterosigmoidostomy
Adrenocortical Excess
    Primary aldosteronism (adenoma or hyperplasia)
    Cushing's syndrome and disease
    Other adrenal steroidal hormone excess
Drug Therapy and Food
    Diuretics
    Licorice
    Adrenal steroids
    Salicylate intoxication
    Outdated tetracycline
Renal Disease (Chronic)
    Potassium-wasting nephropathy
    Nephrotic syndrome
    Renal tubular acidosis
Secondary Hyperaldosteronism
    Renal arterial disease
    Cirrhosis
    Congestive heart failure
Diabetes Mellitus (Acidosis)
Primary Periodic Paralysis
    (Hypokalemic Type)

Routine measurement of serum proteins and hepatic function is usually part of the automated serum chemistry determinations. Although these tests may be of little specific value for the patient with hypertension, they may serve to confirm hemo-concentration (i.e., plasma protein concentration) and provide a baseline for later possible coexisting problems (e.g., myocardial infarction, hepatic diseases). Any pharmacological agent may be incriminated as a causative factor in producing he-patic dysfunction; and, when abnormal hepatic function is detected, it is important to know whether this alteration is related to drug therapy or a coexistent problem. Additionally, alterations in bilirubin metabolism is not an unusual phenomenon (e.g., Gilbert's disease); and it has been of value to know the levels of bilirubin concentrations prior to the initiation of antihypertensive therapy. The thyroid-stimulating hormone (TSH) has been listed in JNC-VI as a useful test in evaluating the patient with hypertension. It is of particular value in suggesting the diagnosis of thyroid disease and in preventing unnecessary evaluation.

Urinary Studies

Of prime importance in the routine urinalysis is the detection of glycosuria for diabetes mellitus; the impaired urine concentration of advancing nephrosclerosis, parenchymal renal disease, and primary aldosteronism; the alkaline urine of primary hyperaldosteronism; and abnormal sediment present in patients with renal parenchymal diseases. Less frequently necessary is a 24-hour urine collection for determining creatinine clearance as well as for assessing dietary sodium intake and potassium wastage. Thus, if the urinary sodium excretion exceeds 100 mEq/24 hr, daily sodium intake is adequate, and there is no dietary factor that would appear to provoke aldosterone stimulation. Moreover, if the urinary excretion of potassium is less than 35 mEq/24 hr, coincident hypokalemia (<3.5 mEq/liter) is less likely to result from excessive adrenal cortical hormone secretion. Conversely, if the 24-hour potassium excretion is excessive (i.e., >50 mEq) in the presence of adequate sodium intake, and there is no other obvious explanation for hypokalemia (<3.5 mEq/liter), there is need to consider hyperaldosteronism or another adrenal steroidal biosynthetic abnormality.

Further, the normal kidney should not excrete more than 200 to 300 mg protein daily. Any amount in excess should suggest parenchymal renal disease (including nephrosclerosis) or an effect of the elevated pressure itself. Nephrosclerosis per se should not provoke protein excretion in excess of 400 to 500 mg daily. However, as suggested, severely elevated arterial pressure may be associated with massive proteinuria; but this should remit with control of arterial pressure. Thus, if urinary protein excretion remains in excess of 400 mg to 500 mg per 24 hours, the physician should consider other causes of renal parenchymal diseases (e.g., glomerulonephritis, renal vein thrombosis). If daily protein excretion exceeds two or three grams, the physician should conclude that chronic pyelonephritis alone is an unlikely cause; a more rational diagnosis should include the various causes of nephrotic syndrome. Microalbuminuria is a more recent (albeit more costly) means of assessing excessive proteinuria more precisely in microquantitative amounts. With current methodology, the normal range for a normal albumin excretion is 30 to 300 mg per day. Urine culture (and sensitivity) is always wise if there is a likelihood of a urinary tract infection or a history of recurrent urinary tract infections.

Chest X-Ray

Although there has been much discussion in recent years on the cost-effectiveness of the routine chest x-ray, it is my opinion that this examination is still of great value in the initial evaluation of any patient, especially one with hypertension. It may be of value in recognizing the presence of left ventricular hypertrophy, but once it is recognized on the x-ray, there is great likelihood that it should be demonstrated electrocardiographically. Most assuredly, it would be shown by the echocardiogram. The physician is reminded of a very useful means for quantifying the degree of cardiac enlargement by determining the Ungerleider index (Figure 2.1). (This technique will provide still more valid information if the films are exposed coincidently with the R wave of the electrocardiogram.) When the Ungerleider Index (that takes into consideration the cardiac size with respect to the patients body habitus) is 15% or more than what would be predicted for that individual, there is a high degree of probability that left ventricular hypertrophy exists. This finding has been derived from studies that correlated the chest films with autopsy findings. There is a great

THEORETIC TRANSVERSE DIAMETERS OF HEART SILHOUETTE FOR VARIOUS HEIGHTS AND WEIGHTS

T D. of Heart	5'0"	1"	2"	3"	4"	5"	6"	7"	8"	9"	10"	11"	6'0"	1"	2"	3"	4"	5"	6"
100 mm	83	85	86	87	89	90	92												
101 "	85	86	88	89	91	92	93	95											
102 "	87	88	90	91	92	94	95	97											
103 "	88	90	92	93	94	96	97	99	100										
104 "	90	92	93	95	96	98	99	101	102										
105 "	92	93	95	96	98	99	101	103	104	106									
106 "	94	95	97	98	100	101	103	104	106	108									
107 "	95	97	99	100	102	103	105	106	108	110	111								
108 "	97	99	100	102	104	105	107	108	110	112	113								
109 "	99	101	102	104	106	107	109	110	112	114	115	117							
110 "	101	102	104	106	108	109	111	113	114	116	118	119	121						
111 "	103	104	106	108	109	111	113	115	116	118	120	121	123	125					
112 "	105	106	108	110	111	113	115	117	118	120	122	124	125	127	129				
113 "	106	108	110	112	113	115	117	119	121	123	124	126	128	129	131	133			
114 "	108	110	112	114	115	117	119	121	123	125	126	128	130	132	133	135	137		
115 "	110	112	114	116	117	119	121	123	125	127	129	130	132	134	136	138	140	141	
116 "	112	114	116	118	120	121	123	125	127	129	131	133	134	136	138	140	142	144	146
117 "	114	116	118	120	122	124	125	127	129	131	133	135	137	139	141	143	144	146	148
118 "	116	118	120	122	124	126	128	129	131	133	135	137	139	141	143	145	147	149	151
119 "	118	120	122	124	126	128	130	132	134	136	138	140	142	143	145	147	149	151	153
120 "	120	122	124	126	128	130	132	134	136	138	140	142	144	146	148	150	152	154	156
121 "	122	124	126	128	130	132	134	136	138	140	142	144	146	148	150	152	154	156	159
122 "	124	126	128	130	132	134	136	138	140	143	145	147	149	151	153	155	157	159	161
123 "	126	128	130	132	134	136	139	141	143	145	147	149	151	153	155	157	160	162	164
124 "	128	130	132	134	137	139	141	143	145	147	149	152	154	156	158	160	162	164	166
125 "	130	132	134	137	139	141	143	145	147	150	152	154	156	158	160	163	165	167	169
126 "	132	134	137	139	141	143	145	148	150	152	154	156	159	161	163	165	167	170	172
127 "	134	137	139	141	143	146	148	150	152	154	157	159	161	163	166	168	170	172	175
128 "	136	139	141	143	146	148	150	152	155	157	159	161	164	166	168	171	173	175	177
129 "	139	141	143	146	148	150	152	155	157	159	162	164	166	169	171	173	176	178	180
130 "	141	143	145	148	150	152	155	157	160	162	164	167	169	171	174	176	178	181	183
131 "	143	145	148	150	152	155	157	160	162	164	167	169	172	174	176	179	181	183	186
132 "	145	148	150	152	155	157	160	162	164	167	169	172	174	177	179	181	184	186	189
133 "	147	150	152	155	157	160	162	165	167	169	172	174	177	179	182	184	187	189	192
134 "	150	152	155	157	160	162	164	167	169	172	174	177	179	182	184	187	189	192	194
135 "	152	154	157	159	162	164	167	169	172	175	177	180	182	185	187	190	192	195	197
136 "	154	157	159	162	164	167	169	172	175	177	180	182	185	187	190	193	195	198	200
137 "	156	159	162	164	167	169	172	175	177	180	182	185	188	190	193	195	198	201	203
138 "	159	161	164	167	169	172	174	177	180	182	185	188	190	193	196	198	201	204	206
139 "	161	164	166	169	172	174	177	180	182	185	188	190	193	196	198	201	204	206	209
140 "	163	166	169	171	174	177	180	182	185	188	190	193	196	199	201	204	207	209	212
141 "	166	168	171	174	177	179	182	185	188	190	193	196	199	201	204	207	210	212	215
142 "	168	171	174	176	179	182	185	188	190	193	196	199	202	204	207	210	213	216	218
143 "	170	173	176	179	182	184	187	190	193	196	199	202	204	207	210	213	216	219	221
144 "	173	176	178	181	184	187	190	193	196	199	201	204	207	210	213	216	219	222	224
145 "	175	178	181	184	187	190	193	196	198	201	204	207	210	213	216	219	222	225	228
146 "	178	180	183	186	189	192	195	198	201	204	207	210	213	216	219	222	225	228	231
147 "	180	183	186	189	192	195	198	201	204	207	210	213	216	219	222	225	228	231	234
148 "	182	185	188	192	195	198	201	204	207	210	213	216	219	222	225	228	231	234	237
149 "	185	188	191	194	197	200	203	206	210	213	216	219	222	225	228	231	234	237	240
150 "	187	191	194	197	200	203	206	209	212	215	219	222	225	228	231	234	237	240	243
151 "	190	193	196	199	203	206	209	212	215	218	222	225	228	231	234	237	241	244	247
152 "	192	196	199	202	205	208	212	215	218	221	224	228	231	234	237	241	244	247	250
153 "	195	198	201	205	208	211	214	218	221	224	227	231	234	237	240	244	247	250	253
154 "	198	201	204	207	211	214	217	221	224	227	230	234	237	240	244	247	250	253	257
155 "	200	203	207	210	213	217	220	224	227	230	233	237	240	243	247	250	253	257	260
156 "		206	210	213	216	220	223	227	230	233	236	240	243	247	250	254	257	260	264
157 "				216	219	222	226	229	233	236	239	243	246	250	253	257	260	263	267
158 "						225	229	232	236	239	243	246	249	253	256	260	263	267	270
159 "								235	239	242	246	249	253	256	260	263	267	270	274
160 "										245	249	252	256	259	263	266	270	274	277
161 "												255	259	263	266	270	273	277	281
162 "												259	262	266	270	273	277	280	284
163 "														269	273	277	280	284	288
164 "														273	276	280	284	287	291

Refer to paper entitled "A Study of the Transverse Diameter of the Heart Silhouette with Prediction Table Based on the Teleoroentgenogram" presented to the Association of Life Insurance Medical Directors of America by Dr. Harry E. Ungerleider of the Equitable Life Assurance Society, and Dr. Charles P. Clark, of the Mutual Benefit Life Insurance Company (1938)

TABLE FOR DETERMINING THE PER CENT. DEVIATION FROM AVERAGE

T D. of Heart	Minus 25%	Minus 20%	Minus 15%	Minus 10%	Minus 5%	Av'ge %	Plus 5%	Plus 10%	Plus 15%	Plus 20%	Plus 25%
100 mm	75	80	85	90	95	100	105	110	115	120	125
101 "	76	81	86	91	96	101	106	111	116	121	126
102 "	77	82	87	92	97	102	107	112	117	122	128
103 "	77	82	88	93	98	103	108	113	118	124	129
104 "	78	83	88	94	99	104	109	114	120	125	130
105 "	79	84	89	95	100	105	110	116	121	126	131
106 "	80	85	90	95	101	106	111	117	122	127	133
107 "	80	86	91	96	102	107	112	118	123	128	134
108 "	81	86	92	97	103	108	113	119	124	130	135
109 "	82	87	93	98	104	109	114	120	125	131	136
110 "	83	88	94	99	105	110	116	121	127	132	138
111 "	83	89	94	100	105	111	117	122	128	133	139
112 "	84	90	95	101	106	112	118	123	129	134	140
113 "	85	90	96	102	107	113	119	124	130	136	141
114 "	86	91	97	103	108	114	120	125	131	137	143
115 "	86	92	98	104	109	115	121	127	132	138	144
116 "	87	93	99	104	110	116	122	128	133	139	145
117 "	88	94	99	105	111	117	123	129	135	140	146
118 "	89	94	100	106	112	118	124	130	136	142	148
119 "	89	95	101	107	113	119	125	131	137	143	149
120 "	90	96	102	108	114	120	126	132	138	144	150
121 "	91	97	103	109	115	121	127	133	139	145	151
122 "	92	98	104	110	116	122	128	134	140	146	153
123 "	92	98	105	111	117	123	129	135	141	148	154
124 "	93	99	105	112	118	124	130	136	143	149	155
125 "	94	100	106	113	119	125	131	138	144	150	156
126 "	95	101	107	113	120	126	132	139	145	151	158
127 "	95	102	108	114	121	127	133	140	146	152	159
128 "	96	102	109	115	122	128	134	141	147	154	160
129 "	97	103	110	116	123	129	135	142	148	155	161
130 "	98	104	111	117	124	130	137	143	150	156	163
131 "	98	105	111	118	124	131	138	144	151	157	164
132 "	99	106	112	119	125	132	139	145	152	158	165
133 "	100	106	113	120	126	133	140	146	153	160	166
134 "	101	107	114	121	127	134	141	147	154	161	168
135 "	101	108	115	122	128	135	142	149	155	162	169
136 "	102	109	116	122	129	136	143	150	156	163	170
137 "	103	110	116	123	130	137	144	151	158	164	171
138 "	104	110	117	124	131	138	145	152	159	166	173
139 "	104	111	118	125	132	139	146	153	160	167	174
140 "	105	112	119	126	133	140	147	154	161	168	175
141 "	106	113	120	127	134	141	148	155	162	169	176
142 "	107	114	121	128	135	142	149	156	163	170	178
143 "	107	114	122	129	136	143	150	157	164	172	179
144 "	108	115	122	130	137	144	151	158	166	173	180
145 "	109	116	123	131	138	145	152	160	167	174	181
146 "	110	117	124	131	139	146	153	161	168	175	183
147 "	110	118	125	132	140	147	154	162	169	176	184
148 "	111	118	126	133	141	148	155	163	170	178	185
149 "	112	119	127	134	142	149	156	164	171	179	186
150 "	113	120	128	135	143	150	158	165	173	180	188
151 "	113	121	128	136	143	151	159	166	174	181	189
152 "	114	122	129	137	144	152	160	167	175	182	190
153 "	115	122	130	138	145	153	161	168	176	184	191
154 "	116	123	131	139	146	154	162	169	177	185	193
155 "	116	124	132	140	147	155	163	171	178	186	194
156 "	117	125	133	140	148	156	164	172	179	187	195
157 "	118	126	133	141	149	157	165	173	181	188	196
158 "	119	126	134	142	150	158	166	174	182	190	198
159 "	119	127	135	143	151	159	167	175	183	191	199
160 "	120	128	136	144	152	160	168	176	184	192	200
161 "	121	129	137	145	153	161	169	177	185	193	201
162 "	122	130	138	146	154	162	170	178	186	194	203
163 "	122	130	139	147	155	163	171	179	187	196	204
164 "	123	131	139	148	156	164	172	180	189	197	205

Figure 2.1. Presentation of tables for deriving the Ungerleider Index from cardiothoracic diameter from the PA chest x-ray and body height and weight.

likelihood of this diagnosis when the index is 10% or more and this is supported further by electrocardiographic indices of left ventricular hypertrophy (*vide infra*).

In addition to its value for detecting the enlarged heart, it is also of value for assessing the stigmata of aortic coarctation (by evidence of costal notching) and, more importantly, as a baseline study for present and future evaluation of pulmonary pathology and the potential later complications from hypertension. (For example, in the follow-up of the long-standing cigarette smoker who did not stop the habit one must periodically look into the possibility of bronchiogenic carcinoma.) When obtained (posteroanteral and left lateral projections), the chest roentgenogram is useful in the foregoing not-infrequent clinical indication and also for the possibility of substernal thyroid, thymoma, and other intrapulmonary or skeletal lesions. In this latter series, let us not forget the value to our patients who insist on smoking and, thereby, incurring the risk of lung cancer.

Electrocardiogram

The primary care and cardiovascular physicians are acutely aware of the necessity for the diagnosis of left ventricular hypertrophy since it is a major independent risk factor. Clearly, this is the diagnostic procedure of choice, and the prior paragraph points to the importance of the chest x-ray itself. The electrocardiogram is of major value for the clinical diagnosis of left ventricular hypertrophy and other abnormalities. If left ventricular hypertrophy is diagnosed by the electrocardiogram in a patient with hypertension (of any Stage of severity), there is little need for performing the echocardiogram (unless there is need for recognizing coexisting cardiac lesions or assessing the stage of ventricular contractility). On the other hand (as will be discussed later), the echocardiogram may be of particular value when there is no evidence of left ventricular hypertrophy by electrocardiogram in patients with Stages I and II hypertension, and cardiac involvement is still suspected. As discussed in the pathophysiological section (chapter 1) and in this chapter under the evaluation of the heart clinically, the electrocardiographic indices of left atrial abnormality are the first signs that can be recognized by chest x-ray or by the electrocardiogram of cardiac involvement from systemic arterial hypertension (Table 2.3). As indicated, this finding provides evidence that the left **ventricle** is already actively adapting to its increased afterload by hypertrophy and is highly concordant with the presence (or absence) of the fourth heart sound (atrial diastolic gallop rhythm or the bruit de galop). As hypertensive heart disease progresses further, left ventricular hypertrophy can be detected by other roentgenographic or electrocardiographic criteria (Table 2.3). Provided in the foregoing are the four criteria for left atrial enlargement; the presence of any two (of the four) is associated with higher systolic and diastolic pressures, a significantly greater chance of obtaining ectopic cardiac beats on a routine 12 lead electrocardiogram, a very high concordance with the atrial diastolic gallop rhythm (fourth heart sound), and echocardiographic evidence of actual atrial enlargement. It goes without saying the electrocardiogram is essential in assessing the patient with cardiac dysrhythmias (which occur more frequently with left ventricular hypertrophy).

Echocardiogram

The echocardiogram is a far greater sensitive means for diagnosing left ventricular hypertrophy. Indeed, many patients with "echo-LVH" may not yet have electrocardiographic evidence of left ventricular hypertrophy. However, it is important to appreciate that the echocardiographic diagnosis of left ventricular hypertrophy, even in its earliest stages, confers a significantly increased risk of premature cardiovascular morbidity and mortality, which is independent of the height of either the systolic or diastolic pressure elevation. In addition to providing the structural evidence of increased left ventricular mass and left ventricular wall thickness (i.e., free wall and septum), the technique also provides important information concerning the function of the heart in hypertension. It is possible to determine atrial (e.g., size and emptying rate) and ventricular (e.g., fiber shortening rate and ejection fraction) function. Patients with atrial enlargement by electrocardiogram have true enlargement of that chamber, and this is associated with an impaired atrial emptying index on echocardiographic study that relates with scintigraphic evidence of impaired ventricular filling. It is clear that the echocardiogram is not indicated for every patient with hypertension. At this time, the electrocardiogram still remains more cost-effective; but this latter statement may be considered controversial by other authorities. Recent reports suggest that a **limited echocardiogram** (employing only M-mode indices) may be more cost-effective than the M-Mode, 2-D Doppler echocardiogram when only left ventricular hypertrophy must be detected. In my personal experience, however, I find that the echocardiogram is of particular value when the diagnosis of left ventricular hypertrophy or the functional status of the left ventricle is of importance clinically, when one is interested in learning about the progression of cardiac involvement in a patient with hypertensive heart disease, when there is a question as to the structural or functional effect of antihypertensive drug therapy and, of course, for the myriad of other indications and needs that this important diagnostic technique provides. In general, there are no murmurs that are related to hypertensive heart disease although, in patients with severely elevated arterial hypertension, the aortic diastolic murmur of aortic insufficiency may appear associated with the eversion of the aortic cusp by the increased ventricular afterload. An excellent documentation of this now rare finding (with the advent of effective antihypertensive therapy) may be found in the earlier editions of Levine and Harvey's textbook on auscultation. Of interest is the disappearance of this "functional" murmur coincident with reduction of pressure even contemporaneously with pressure reduction using intravenous sodium nitroprusside. A functional and idiopathic mitral valvular prolapse syndrome has been documented in patients with borderline and mild essential hypertension associated with a hyperdynamic beta-adrenergic circulatory state. This alteration has been associated with the mitral click, echocardiographic evidence of prolapsed posterior leaflet of the mitral valve, elevated circulating levels of norepinephrine, and increased responsiveness to the pharmacological beta-adrenergic receptor agonist isoproterenol.

OTHER LABORATORY STUDIES

Although they are clearly not indicated in all patients with uncomplicated essential hypertension (by far the vast majority of patients with hypertension), a number of older and newer studies are available to assess etiology or complications from hypertension (Table 2.6). The following discussion includes information which may be of value for the cardiovascular physician, internist, or other primary care provider in some of these tests. (The first discussion concerning nuclear imaging is provided because it follows naturally from the prior discussion on cardiac assessment.)

Table 2.6. Other Laboratory Studies of Possible Value in the Diagnostic Evaluation of Patients with Hypertension.

*Chest x-ray (PA and lateral projections)
*Electrocardiogram (12 lead, conventional)
Intravenous urogram ("hypertensive IVP")
Renal arteriography
Bilateral renal venous renin determinations
Isotope renography and renal scans
Thyroid function studies
Plasma parahormone concentration
Blood volume determination (plasma volume, RBC mass)
Radioimmunoassay studies
   Plasma renin activity
   Plasma angiotensin I or II or angiotensin-converting enzyme levels
   Plasma aldosterone level
   Human growth hormone levels
   Plasma insulin levels
Urinary hormone excretion studies (24-hour collection)
   Catecholamines, VMA, metanephrines concentration in urine
   Plasma catecholamine levels
   Plasma aldosterone levels
   Corticosteroids and ketosteroids
Clonidine suppression test for pheochromocytoma (see Chapter 4)

Not all of these studies are deemed necessary; those with strong necessity (from the author's viewpoint) are marked with an asterisk (*)

Nuclear Imaging

Myocardial scintigraphic scanning using any of several radioisotopic modalities, is of importance in assessing cardiac function as well as for obtaining some index of the perfusion of the left ventricle, particularly when myocardial ischemia is of concern. Thus, in the patient with left ventricular hypertrophy associated with cardiac dysrhythmias or with treadmill abnormalities suggesting ischemic heart disease the nuclear scan can be of great help. It is important to appreciate, however, that a normal thallium scan in a patient with hypertensive heart disease neither fully excludes the diagnosis of obstructive epicardial disease nor even the additional likelihood of small vessel arteriolar disease in the patient with hypertensive heart disease having evidence of "silent ischemia" or so-called "microvascular angina." In recent years, the thallium scan has not been adequate (especially in the latter patients), and some index of coronary vascular reserve is of value. This may be provided by employing thallium scintigraphy before and after pharmacologically induced coronary vasodilation (e.g., with dipyridamole, adenosine). This is an area of intensive investigation at this time; also being evaluated are the use of technetium cistamebi and other nuclear methods. But, until more experience is obtained, it is wise to realize that, at present, none of the reports have systematically provided their broad pharmacological evaluation using dose-response relationships or have provided data involving repeated findings in the same patient and under similar conditions. Also advocated by some are magnetic resonance imaging and positron emission technology for evaluating left ventricular hypertrophy but, at this time, their clinical applicability must still be demonstrated.

Intravenous Urography

In general, it is not necessary to perform routine intravenous urography (IVP) to evaluate every patient with essential hypertension. However, the study is of value if the patient with hypertension is a child or adolescent, young woman, or a patient who was hypertensive during pregnancy and has remained so postpartum; there is no family history of hypertension; there is sudden worsening of the hypertensive disease; if there is a past or present history of renal parenchymal disease; or if the diagnosis of renal arterial disease has been established and the patient is being followed for progression of the disease. However, to my way of thinking, if renal arterial disease is strongly suggested or definitive diagnosis is necessary, I would proceed directly to the performance of selective renal arteriography with differential renal venous renin determinations. It is also helpful to request that the radiologist obtain a postarteriographic flat plate of the abdomen to determine the renal excretory findings as the arteriographic contrast material is being excreted from the kidney. It is important to measure the renal sizes (including the lengths and widths of each kidney) and tabulate these data in the patient's record, representing the average of several film measurements. In general, the right kidney may be from 0.5 to 1.0 cm shorter than the left, so that if the left kidney is 0.5 to 1.0 cm shorter than the right there may be a greater likelihood of potential renal arterial occlusive disease of the left kidney. Furthermore, if there is any evidence of delay in the appearance of contrast material in one kidney, if there is significant disparity of renal lengths (as indicated), or if there is any evidence of lack of segmental renal function, then there is sufficient justification to proceed with selective renal arteriography.

One should remember that performance of intravenous urography is not by any means the exclusive reason for progressing to arteriography (Table 2.7). Thus, if renal arterial disease is a strong consideration, it may be wise and more cost-effective to obtain selective renal arteriography at the outset. Conversely, the potential diagnosis of renal arterial disease is not the major indication for intravenous urography. More common is the consideration to determine whether there is evidence of renal parenchymal disease, and this includes the early and more subtle findings of chronic pyelonephritis. The physician must remember that prior to the development of chronic renal failure, there must be earlier evidence of renal parenchymal disease, and if we are to prevent progression of renal functional impairment, we must vigorously search for the earliest renal findings.

Selective Renal Arteriography

Several years ago I was told that if renal arterial disease is to be diagnosed at all, one must be prepared to visualize the renal arteries. This very obvious truth frequently is not realized by physicians who seem more committed to establishing the presence of renal arterial disease by other less specific and more indirect methods. Thus, for many years definition of significant renal arterial disease was based on findings of impaired renal excretory function. It may be more reasonable to relate "significance" in terms of its pressor implications; then one should find a means to quantify the renal pressor alteration of the arterial lesion. This has been made feasible with the de-

Table 2.7. Specialized Studies of Value in Evaluating Patients with Hypertension Suspected as Having Renal Arterial Disease.*

Study	Indications
Intravenous urography	Consideration of renal parenchymal disease. History of urinary tract infections, renal stones, or obstructive uropathy. Persistence of hypertension after toxemia of pregnancy.
Selective renal arteriography (May be preceded by digital subtraction angiography in outpatients)	Abdominal, flank, or back bruit (see text). Sudden onset of hypertension. Sudden severity of known hypertension, including loss of blood pressure control on previously adequate therapy. Disparity in renal lengths (by urography or scintigraphy) of ≥1 cm.
Renal venous renin activities	Functional assessment of the arterial lesion(s) at the time of selective renal arteriography. Possible outpatient use after digital subtraction arteriograms have demonstrated arterial disease. Evaluation of progression of known renal arterial disease.
Isotope renography and renal scans	Follow-up of patient with diagnosed renal arterial disease (e.g., to assess reduction in renal size or to compare postoperative to preoperative studies). Postoperative assessment of the patency of renal blood supply. Use in conjunction with digital subtraction arteriography. Confirmation of clinical suspicion of renal arterial lesion on patient allergic to contrast material in order to obviate steroidal preparation of patient for arteriographic study.
Plasma renin activity (Peripheral venous blood)	Assessment of low-renin forms of hypertension (e.g., primary aldosteronism, volume-dependent hypertension). Assessment of high-renin forms of hypertension (renal arterial disease or high-renin essential hypertension). Captopril renography or with renal artery ultrasound has been introduced for diagnostic assessment of renal arterial disease. At present the ultimate utility for these studies remains to be defined.

*These studies are indicated if a specific cause of hypertension is considered or if target organ involvement and other complications of the disease are suspected.

termination of plasma renal venous renin determinations. Thus, if the ratio of plasma renin activity of the affected to the unaffected kidney in renal venous blood is 1.6 or more, there is further reason to ascribe true significance to the renal arterial lesion. Other studies in this respect include the captopril renogram with or without renal artery ultrasound.

An additional consideration must be the pathologic nature of the renal arterial lesion. In this regard, the physician must realize that considerable information is available to suggest not only the significance but also the natural history of the disease from the arteriographic findings. For example, if the renal mass is severely contracted, the implication is that the lesion must be "significant."

There are basically two types of renal arterial disease: the atherosclerotic and the nonatherosclerotic (or fibrosing) lesion. With respect to the former, hypertension may have preceded the development of the lesion (e.g., hypertension may facilitate the progression of atherosclerosis) or it may be the result of the arterial lesion (e.g., renovascular hypertension). With respect to the probable response to corrective surgery in these patients with atherosclerotic plaques (and in patients with segmental lesions), much assistance may be provided by renal venous renin studies. Thus, if there is no evidence of increased production of renin by the "affected" kidney—especially if the affected kidney is not contracted in size—it might be wiser to treat the patient pharmacologically and to follow that patient with periodic radiographic or isotopic studies (e.g., intravenous urography, renal scans, or isotope renograms). If, on the other hand, renal parenchymal function seems to be deteriorating (as evidenced by further diminution of renal size or if the pressure becomes increasingly more difficult to control), surgical measures might be indicated. In any event, the physician should realize that atherosclerotic renal arterial disease is part of a much broader systemic vascular disease, and prior to any surgical procedure the patient should be evaluated for atherosclerotic vascular disease involving the coronary, cerebral, mesenteric, and great vessels.

There are several types of the other form of renal arterial disease (i.e., fibrosing disease). Not infrequently, these patients present no family history of hypertension, but a renal arterial bruit may be audible over the abdomen or flanks. In these patients there is a higher probability that surgical correction of these lesions might be expected to be associated with a normalization of arterial pressures. In some of these patients, involvement of both renal arteries may be present; this is found most often with the "string of beads" type of lesion, also termed *perimedial fibroplasia.* Fortunately, this type of lesion progresses relatively slowly, is one of the most common of the fibrosing lesions, and the associated elevated blood pressure may be treated pharmacologically while the patient is periodically observed for evidence of progression of the arterial disease. There are several other types of fibrosing renal arterial disease, and these seem to be more likely to progress in severity. These types of renal arterial disease may be complicated by aneurysm formation, dissection, and thrombosis of the renal artery. For these reasons, surgical treatment may be considered more urgent; but, in any event, the general physical condition of the patient should be considered. (For a more detailed discussion concerning the diagnosis, treatment, and varieties of renal arterial disease and hypertension, the reader is referred to Chapter 8 and other more specific references.)

Renal Venous Renin Determinations

We already have alluded to the importance of these findings in interpreting the significance of renal arterial disease, particularly in the patient with atherosclerotic and bilateral renal arterial disease. However, after many years of use, I am still not yet fully convinced that inability to demonstrate a specific ratio of renal venous renin activity means that surgical treatment will be unsuccessful. A sufficient number of patients with so-called "normal" ratios have not been subjected to surgery and analyzed to determine whether the elevated arterial pressure might have been corrected had surgery been performed. With respect to another caution, physicians have pursued the collection of their renin data differently. Some insist that their patient not have any pharmacologic therapy prior to renal venous renin collections, and others insist that their patients be treated with a stimulating dose of a diuretic of one type or another or an angiotensin-converting enzyme inhibitor. At present, however, many authorities employ the captopril stimulation test (using 25 or 50 mg of the drug). A positive test is one in which the plasma renin activity is at least 150 percent greater than the pre-captopril administration level. To confuse this problem further, many physicians obtain renal venous renins while their patients receive a variety of antihypertensive (and other) drugs that may suppress or stimulate plasma renin activity. It therefore seems valid for us to ask the following questions: First, how does premedication (for arteriography) affect the results? Second, how does prior introduction of radiocontrast material into the renal artery (it affects intrarenal hemodynamics) affect renin release? Third, if a patient is receiving antihypertensive therapy, how does this affect the release of renin by the affected and unaffected kidneys? Fourth, do the affected and unaffected kidneys respond similarly to the same doses of antihypertensive drugs, and how does this affect the release of renin by the affected and unaffected kidneys? Fifth, if these kidneys respond differently, what is the significance of the stimulation tests using low-sodium diet and diuretics of varying types? The answers to these questions are still not yet completely available; we must await this information, but we must also realize that our understanding of the problem has improved vastly in recent years.

Isotope Renography and Renal Scans

Reference to these studies already has been made. Their greatest value, may be related to the follow-up care of a patient with renal arterial disease once diagnosis has been made. Thus, if a renal arterial lesion has been demonstrated and the physician and patient elect to pursue pharmacologic treatment and to observe for progression of the disease, these noninvasive isotopic studies might provide evidence of further contraction of the renal mass and delay in appearance of the isotope to the kidney. In addition, these studies may be useful if surgical correction of the arterial lesion is elected. Then it might be wise to obtain preoperative studies in order to measure changes in appearance of isotope and change in renal mass during the immediate postoperative period. Thus, if vascular surgery is performed and the physician is interested in learning whether patency of the artery or graft is maintained in the early postoperative period (when arterial pressure either has not fallen or has increased further), and if renal arteriography is considered too hazardous, the isotopic renogram or scan may be of extreme value. Finally, isotopic renography has been utilized more recently before and after the oral administration of a single dose of captopril, an angiotensin-converting enzyme inhibitor to assess the potential participation of a renal arterial lesion in reducing renal blood flow of an affected kidney. The drug has also been used in conjunction with renal ultrasonography for renal arterial stenosis. In either case, the ultimate utility of the study has not yet been fully resolved.

Plasma Renin Activity

Without entering into the dialogue of the current controversy of the role of plasma renin activity in current medical practice, a few words seem indicated to permit interpretation of these tests. First, the physician must have confidence in the laboratory he uses for measurement of PRA (the common term for the test). Second, he must be aware of the pitfalls in collection; and, third, he must be aware of the physiologic implications of the results. The physician must be aware of the many drugs and physiologic conditions that alter plasma renin activity. For example, upright posture, exercise, time of day, diuretic therapy, vasodilators, angiotensin-converting enzyme inhibitors, recent blood donation, oral contraceptives, and anesthetic agents all will increase plasma renin activity. Moreover, permitting the withdrawn blood sample to stand at room temperature, failure to centrifuge the blood immediately in a cold centrifuge (thereby permitting plasma angiotensinase to act on the blood), and adrenolytic therapy (including beta-adrenergic blocking drugs) all reduce plasma renin activity. And, since plasma renin activity increases with contraction of intravascular volume, this factor also is important in interpretation of the results. Therefore, it is not surprising that the patient with high arterial pressure and severely contracted intravascular volume (e.g., malignant hypertension) will have a high plasma renin activity and that the patient with volume-dependent hypertension (e.g., primary aldosteronism) will exhibit low plasma renin activity. It therefore follows (with respect to the concept of specificity of antihypertensive therapy) that the patient with low renin essential hypertension (or volume-dependent essential hypertension) will also respond to volume contraction (i.e., diuretic therapy) and the patient with high plasma renin essential hypertension will respond to adrenergic suppression. Indeed, these concepts provide the basis for the presently debated therapeutic and pathogenetic concepts.

Hormonal Studies

With the introduction of radioimmunoassay technology, the means for the diagnosis of a variety of hormonal types of hypertension are available (Table 2.6). Already we have seen the usefulness of the measurement of plasma renin activity and aldosterone in plasma. Other immunoassay measurements include that of insulin and growth hormone. In addition, measurement of blood thyroid hormonal functions, parahormone, and catecholamines are available. Moreover, urinary determination of excretion rates of catecholamines (and their metabolites), aldosterone, and other adrenal steroids are well established. For a more detailed discussion concerning the more specialized hormonal studies, the reader is referred to more specialized textbook of endocrinology.

Ambulatory Pressure Monitoring

Another controversially employed diagnostic technique is that of 24-hour ambulatory sphygmomanometry. This technique is particularly useful when there is some question existing between the office blood pressure measurements and cardiac findings (e.g, size, wall thickness, and function) and height of pressure. Other clinical situations that may indicate usefulness of this technology might be related to nocturnal angina or in the patient with "spells" suggesting orthostatic hypotension under usual activities. (Table 2.8 details further indications for 24 hours-or-less ambulatory blood pressure recording.) Still other situations may be related to associated Holter electrocardiographic monitoring and evaluation of hypertensive heart disease or for ascertaining the effects of a specific antihypertensive treatment program. Other authorities have employed this technology for determining the pressures during daily

Table 2.8. Indications for Automated Blood Pressure Recording.

1. To confirm office blood pressure readings (e.g., office or white coat hypertension).
2. To determine variability of blood pressures during 24-hour period.
3. For patients with systemic hypertension and "spells" with suspected pheochromocytoma, episodic hypertension, or similar diagnoses.
4. To evaluate hypotensive symptoms associated with antihypertensive medications or autonomic dysfunction.
5. To relate blood pressure elevation with episodes of angina pectoris or other cardiac symptoms.
6. To determine whether nocturnal angina is related to blood pressure elevation.
7. To evaluate carotid sinus syncope or pacemaker syndromes (together with Holter electrocardiographic monitoring).
8. To provide confirmation that blood pressure is well controlled and that antihypertensive treatment is efficacious.
9. To evaluate antihypertensive drug resistance.
10. To determine whether blood pressures may be elevated when office blood pressures and when target organ involvement (e.g., of heart, kidneys, and brain) are abnormal.
11. To support insurance or other "third party" needs demonstrating control (or lack of control) of blood pressure levels.
12. For research purposes.

activities in patients suspected as having so-called "office" or "white-coat" hypertension. With respect to the latter popular and controversial subject, it is my personal opinion that the technique is, at present, too expensive for routine use and that sufficient normative data are not yet available to define what normal prognostic data concerning risk associated with blood pressure ambulatory pressures really are. Moreover, all existing measurements presently relate to repeated measurements of casual pressures taken in the office setting. Whether pressures may be lower during daily activity has not been related to prognosis epidemiologically. In the final analysis, home blood pressure measurements and records have been found to be useful and cheaper. In this regard, I personally recommend the use of mercury sphygmomanometry (by another familial observer) or aneroid devices that are calibratable (several models can be inflated and deflated by the patient while listening to the sounds and visualizing the pressure gauge) rather than the newer electronic and non-calibrated devices. To this end, aneroid instruments with an attachable stethoscope to the cuff itself are extremely reliable as easily purchased or may be purchased through local medical supply stores.

PERSONAL VIEWPOINT ON "WHITE COAT HYPERTENSION" AND HOME BLOOD PRESSURE MEASUREMENT

There is no doubt that blood pressure measurements obtained in the physician's office or other health care settings may be higher than pressures that are taken by the patients at home or in other settings as well as by automatic portable blood pressure measuring devices. For this reason, I frequently instruct patients in taking their own pressures at home and report these pressures (taken regularly at the same time using the same procedure). These records are valuable in deciding the questions concerning whether the elevated pressure should be reduced with antihypertensive drugs and in arriving at an effective treatment program. Personally, I prefer the patients to use mercury sphygmomanometers (usually employed by another family member) or an aneroid "cuff" in which the bulb and manometer are in a single entity that is attached to the cuff and can be held and inflated by the contralateral hand. These instruments are all calibratable in contrast to the less reliable electronic devices (in my opinion).

Patients with higher pressures in the office setting with "normal" pressures at home are said to have "white coat hypertension." In these patients, home pressures are extremely useful, although some physicians also employ ambulatory and automatic devices which are, obviously, more costly and must be employed with some judgment. Just what is correct, office versus automatic pressures, continues to be an issue of ongoing controversy. In my opinion, the 24-hour ambulatory pressures cannot define a truly normal pressure since, at present, there are inadequate normative data for individuals of all ages, both genders, and all races. Moreover, all epidemiological actuarial data are based on the "casual" pressures that have been obtained in the office setting in millions of patients (for third party insurers). Hence, the issue of whether the patient with "white coat hypertension" is normal or "hypertensive" remains to be defined. Until then, I believe there are definite rules for 24-hour (or less) ambulatory pressures and are presented in Table 2.8.

REFERENCES

1. Joint National Committee on Detection, Evaluation, and Treatment of High Blood Pressure: The 1992 Report of the Joint National Committee on Detection, Evaluation, and Treatment of High Blood Pressure (JNC-VI). Arch Intern Med 1997; 157:2413–2446.
2. Frohlich ED. Evaluation and management of the patient with essential hypertension. In: Cardiology (Parmley WW, Chaterjee K, eds.). JB Lippincott, Philadelphia, 1994, pp. 1–17.
   The above two papers present a more detailed discussion on the initial evaluation of the patient with hypertension.
3. Oren S, Grossman E, Messerli FH, Frohlich ED. High blood pressure: Side-effects of drugs, poisons, and food. Cardiol Clin 1988; 6:467–474.
   The reference presents a detailed discussion of the variety of agents that may exacerbate an elevation in arterial pressure, particularly in a patient with hypertension.
4. Keith NM, Wagener HP, Barker NN. Some different types of essential hypertension: Their course and prognosis. Am J Med Sci 1939, 197:332.
   The classical article detailing the classification of hypertensive retinopathy.
5. Wagener HP, Clay GE, Gipner JF. Classification of retinal lesions in presence of vascular hypertension: Report submitted by committee. Trans Am Ophthalmol Soc 1947; 45:57.
   A different presentation of the graduations of severity of hypertensive retinopathy from the more specialized concept of the ophthalmologist.

6. Chrysanthakopoulos SG, Frohlich ED, Adamopoulos PN, et al. The pathophysiologic significance of "stress polycythemia" in essential hypertension. Am J Cardiol 1976; 37:1069–1072.
A discussion of the underlying mechanisms associated with polycythemia in patients with hypertensive disease.

7. Ungerleider HE, Clark CP. Study of the transverse diameter of the heart silhouette with prediction table based on the teleroentgenogram. Am Heart J 1939; 17:92.
The original presentation of the relationship of chest x-ray evidence of left ventricular hypertrophy to anatomical evidence of cardiac enlargement in hypertension.

8. Tarazi RC, Miller A, Frohlich ED, Dustan HP. Electrocardiographic changes reflecting left atrial abnormality in hypertension. Circulation, 1966; 34:818–822.

9. Messerli FH, Frohlich ED, Dreslinski GR et al. Serum uric acid in essential hypertension: An indicator of renal vascular involvement. Ann Intern Med 1980; 93:817–821.

10. Frohlich ED. Classic Papers Symposium: History of Medicine Series: Surrogate indexes of target organ involvement in hypertension. Am J Med Sci 1996; 312:225–228.

11. Frohlich ED, Re RN. Pathophysiology of Systemic Arterial Hypertension. In: Hurst's The Heart, 9th edition. Editors: Alexander RW, Schlant RC, Fuster V, O'Rourke RA, Roberts R, Sonnenblick EH, The McGraw-Hill Companies, New York 1998, pp. 1635-1650.

12. Hall DW. Diagnostic evaluation of the patient with systemic arterial hypertension. In: Hurst's The Heart, 9th edition. Editors: Alexander RW, Schlant RC, Fuster V, O'Rourke RA, Roberts R, Sonnenblick EH, The McGraw-Hill Companies, New York 1998, pp. 1651–1672.
The above five references provide the background for the surrogate indices of early target organ involvement of heart and kidney from hypertensive disease.

13. Sheps SG, Frohlich ED. Limited Echocardiography for Hypertensive Left Ventricular Hypertrophy. An Opinion Statement. Hypertension 1997; 29:560–563.
This is the first paper providing data and recommendations for clinical outcomes of echocardiography in patients with hypertension and for use of a more limited and cost effective echocardiographic.

SECTION II

ANTIHYPERTENSIVE THERAPY

Chapter 3

Historical and Lifestyle Modification Concepts

As indicated in the Acknowledgments at the beginning of this book, the field of hypertension has enjoyed tremendous progress and growth over the past four decades. No facet of this broad area of inquiry and clinical practice has contributed more to the overall changes in this field and in cardiovascular medicine, in general, than in the area of therapeutics. With these outstanding advances in therapies, remarkably innovative concepts dealing with the underlying mechanisms of disease have evolved. Still more exciting, these new pharmacological advances have made major novel contributions to other areas of medicine.

Along the way, many concepts of antihypertensive therapy have been surrounded by controversy, debate, resolution, and more controversy. This section of the book details the present status of antihypertensive therapy; other chapters in this book will also encompass some of the current debates and will focus upon many aspects of hypertensive disease and their treatments. For the more specific details on the treatment of special populations of hypertensive patients, the reader is referred to the next section of this book. Much has been resolved over the years concerning the following: the wisdom of reducing arterial pressure; role of nonpharmacologic approaches to treatment; merits and applicability of the various classes of antihypertensive agents; mechanisms of action of each drug class; clinical goals of antihypertensive therapy; selection of antihypertensive therapeutic agents; and other issues. Notwithstanding many of these unresolved issues, this remarkable therapeutic revolution and evolution continues to provide an ongoing story of successes in the reduction of cardiovascular morbidity and mortality related to the hypertensive and other cardiovascular, endocrine, neurological, and renal diseases.

BRIEF HISTORICAL PERSPECTIVE

It was four decades ago, in the mid-1950s, that hypertension was just becoming perceived as a disease associated with premature morbidity and mortality requiring treatment. Adequate therapy was still unavailable. Indeed, the medical profession had just begun to appreciate that there was nothing truly "essential" to the diagnosis of essential hypertension other than the essential need to understand more about the disease mechanisms and to control severely elevated arterial pressure. The United States had just emerged from World War II and its national leader, Franklin D. Roosevelt, had died suddenly from a cerebral hemorrhage secondary to long-standing uncontrolled hypertension. The picture of this rapidly aging man on his return from the Yalta Conference remains etched into history. It is still difficult to believe that this man was only 63 years of age, less than two years younger than his more youthful appearing successor, Harry

S Truman. As another independent observation, many of the young men recruited into the military in that war, who were told their blood pressures were slightly elevated at their initial selective service physical examination was the result of situational anxiety, were soon to appear at the Veterans Administration Hospitals with target organ consequences of hypertensive disease: congestive heart failure; accelerated and malignant hypertension or other hypertensive emergencies; angina pectoris and myocardial infarction; dissecting aortic aneurysm; thrombotic and hemorrhagic strokes; and, even more recently, renal functional impairment and failure.

The management of hypertension in those earlier days of the 1940s—phenobarbital, rest, and the "pyrogen therapies"—were becoming recognized for what they were: ineffective or of no value whatsoever. Appearing to be more useful were the age-old concept of sodium restriction and the rice-fruit diet, new surgical approaches (i.e., thoracodorsal sympathectomy with or without bilateral adrenalectomy), and the newer and very potent pharmacotherapeutical agents. The latter two forms of treatment were becoming notorious for their lack of predictability and their bothersome side effects, respectively. The ganglion-blocking agents were associated with severe postural hypotension, paralytic ileus, severe constipation, impotency, visual disturbances, and pulmonary fibrosis. Notwithstanding these major problems, patients receiving these drugs were demonstrating reversal of the natural history and the pathological consequences of the disease as arterial pressure was controlled. Indeed, these treatments were becoming so impressive that patients with malignant hypertension demonstrated regression of the exudative retinopathy and reversal of papilledema associated with hypertensive retinopathy with control of arterial pressure. Most important, these patients were living longer. Thus, prior to these treatments, 97 percent of these patients died within three months.

By the late 1950s, new classes of antihypertensive agents were being introduced on a regular basis. First, there were the veratrum alkaloids; they reduced arterial pressure effectively, but treatment was complicated by a very narrow therapeutic index manifested by nausea and vomiting that was closely associated with effective pressure reduction. The direct-acting vascular smooth muscle relaxant and vasodilator hydralazine was introduced and found to be effective parenterally in patients with hypertensive emergencies as well as in patients with less severe disease when the oral formulation was used. But soon, however, a lupus erythematosus-like syndrome was found to occur in those patients receiving higher doses (400 mg/day and more). Reserpine and the other rauwolfia alkaloids were also found to be effective in reducing pressure for patients with severe disease using injectable doses and for others with less severe disease using lower oral doses. However, it was not until the thiazide diuretics were introduced by the end of the 1950s that antihypertensive therapy was shown to be feasible on a broad scale for more widespread use by the primary care physician. Each of the available antihypertensive drug classes were rendered even more efficacious and safe with the addition of the orally administered thiazide diuretic. Furthermore, not only could these agents be used alone with significant control of blood pressure in a certain number of patients with hypertension, but it was soon learned that these agents could be employed synergistically with the diuretics and other antihypertensive drug classes. Indeed, by combination, it was possible to use the other classes of drugs in smaller doses and with less attendant side effects.

This efficacy of antihypertensive therapy received its greatest impetus following the publication of the initial results by the first multicenter, placebo-controlled trials of the Veterans Administration Cooperative Study. Using the foregoing concept that the thiazides could reduce pressure predictably in a high percentage of patients with essential hypertension, and that its effectiveness could enhance the hypotensive effects of reserpine and hydralazine when sequentially added in lower doses than when each was used alone, the so-called "stepped-care" algorithm approach to antihypertensive therapy was introduced by the Veterans Administration. These reports were soon reinforced by other multicenter controlled trials worldwide from U.S. Public Health Service, Medical Research Council trials in Great Britain, and others from Sweden, Norway, Australia, and other countries. They all demonstrated conclusively the efficacy of antihypertensive therapy and that this approach to treatment would also be associated with a definite reduction in the morbidity and mortality from hypertension and its complications as well as from other cardiovascular diseases. For this remarkably new approach, Edward D. Freis, M.D., received the Lasker Award, providing recognition of this new therapeutic advance and the impetus for the establishment of a National High Blood Pressure Education Program that has been the paradigm for other national high blood pressure programs worldwide.

Since those earlier days, a large series of other multicenter controlled trials ensued that were sponsored by the National Heart Lung and Blood Institute in the United States (e.g., Hypertension Detection and Follow-Up Program, Multiple Risk Factor Intervention Trial, Treatment of Mild Hypertension, and others), Medical Research Council in Great Britain, European Working Party in Elderly Hypertension, and studies from Australia, Sweden, and other nations. Their results continued to support the rationale, feasibility, and necessity for controlling elevated arterial pressure at lower (below 90 mmHg) diastolic pressure levels. More recently, other trials, conducted in more sophisticated fashions worldwide, demonstrated the efficacy of controlling systolic as well as diastolic pressure elevations. And, at the present time, a number of other protocols are in progress for other specialized groups of hypertensive populations. These results have led to the current recommendations in JNC-VI, that goal blood pressures, therapeutically, should be set to less than 140 and 90 mm Hg for systolic and diastolic pressures, respectively, all factors being equal.

At present, the number of classes of antihypertensive agents continues to increase, providing a greater spectrum of drug actions and a broader means for suppressing a myriad of additional pressor mechanisms that subserve the maintenance of elevated pressure in patients with hypertensive diseases. Amazing new agents and antihypertensive drug classes attest to the scientific imagination and ability of the pharmaceutical industry and the means to stimulate the intellectual inquiry by fundamental and clinical scientists to understand in greater depth the underlying disease mechanisms of hypertension. The mechanisms of these new classes of antihypertensive drugs have become more sophisticated, demonstrating inhibition of newer and more challenging pressor mechanisms (Table 3.1). Some of these classes of agents have already been introduced (e.g., angiotensin II receptor antagonists, serotonin inhibitors, specific inhibitors of prostoglandins), others are in trial at this time (e.g., renin inhibitors, bradykinin antagonists, potassium channel agonists, aminopeptidase inhibitors that diminish the metabolism of atrial natriuretic factor, vasopressin antagonists, dopamine receptor stimulators and inhibitors), and still others are yet newer in concept and in action.

THE "IDEAL" AGENT

Clearly, any agent that is suitable for the treatment of hypertension must have the intrinsic ability to antagonize the hemodynamic alterations that characterize that form of clinical hypertension. Hence, they should be able to reduce arterial pressure through a

Table 3.1. Drug Classes Under Current Study and Trials.

- Angiotensin II receptor antagonists
- Serotonin antagonists
- Dopamine receptor agonists
- Renin inhibitors
- Potassium channel activators
- Neutral endopeptidase inhibitors
- Vasopressin antagonists
- Agents interacting on kinin system
- Agents interacting with prostaglandin system

reduction of the total peripheral resistance and the component organ vascular resistances that seem to be uniformly increased in most forms of clinical hypertension. They should achieve these effects with minimal reflex cardiac stimulation so that heart rate, cardiac output, myocardial contractility, and myocardial oxygen demand are not increased. For example, cardiac stimulation by an antihypertensive agent (either directly or reflexively) in a patient with occlusive epicardial coronary artery disease, cardiac failure, or dissecting aortic aneurysm may precipitate angina pectoris or myocardial infarction, exacerbate cardiac failure, and enhance aortic dissection, respectively. Moreover, in response to the reduction in hydrostatic and renal perfusion pressures, intravascular volume should not expand. In the earlier days of antihypertensive therapy, the reduction in arterial pressure and vascular resistance associated with the adrenergic inhibitors and the direct-acting vasodilators were associated with an expanded intravascular volume that attenuated the fall in pressure (i.e., the "pseudotolerance" phenomenon). In addition, associated with the achieved reduction in arterial pressure and total and regional vascular resistances, cardiac output and blood flow to the major organs (particularly to heart, kidneys, and brain) should be maintained in order that organ function would not deteriorate further and, preferably, might even improve. Furthermore, the agents should be able to reverse the structural changes and increased independent risk associated with these changes. At the present time, reversal of these structural alterations have been demonstrated experimentally and clinically, but these reversed structural changes have not yet been shown to reduce that associated risk.

In addition to these important physiological actions, the agent should not produce significant adverse effects. Ideally, the drug should be able to work alone as monotherapy, should be administered preferably only once daily, and should be inexpensive. Should the drug be less than optimally effective in controlling arterial pressure, it should be compatible with the other widely prescribed antihypertensive agents without producing drug interactions but, hopefully, in synergy with their mutual antihypertensive benefits.

Having described this "shopping list" for an ideal antihypertensive agent, we should acknowledge the fact that no agent thus far developed has achieved all of these goals. However, many of the newer agents seem to be approaching it, and no one agent probably can be considered the "ideal" for all patients with hypertension (Table 3.2).

NONPHARMACOLOGICAL THERAPY/LIFESTYLE MODIFICATIONS

The importance of nonpharmacologic therapy of hypertension was first introduced in the third Joint National Committee's report on the detection, evaluation, and treatment of hypertension and in a more expanded document published shortly thereafter.

TABLE 3.2. Properties of an "Ideal" Antihypertensive Agent.

1. It antagonizes the hemodynamic alterations that characterize hypertension.
2. It produces pressure reduction without reflex cardiac stimulation.
3. Pressure reduction should not promote "pseudotolerance."
4. Maintenance of cardiac output and regional blood flows to major organs.
5. It reverses structural alterations and the intrinsic risk associated with these changes.
6. It has minimal adverse effects.
7. It is useful as a monotherapeutic agent.
8. It is compatible with other widely used antihypertensive agents.
9. It is inexpensive.

At that time, the only measures recommended were weight control, sodium restriction, and moderation of alcohol intake. Other measures including dietary restriction of animal fat intake, cessation of cigarette smoking, and incorporation of a routine exercise program into one's lifestyle were noted as important health measures for overall good cardiovascular health. These nonpharmacological interventions for the treatment of hypertension were considered valuable since it was held that those patients with what was then termed "mild hypertension" (particularly those whose diastolic pressures fell between 90 and 94 mmHg) might demonstrate blood pressure reduction without the need for drug therapy. It was also suggested that if these were continued—even in patients with more severe levels of diastolic hypertension—they may also impart significant antihypertensive benefits to other patients. Thus, there was sufficient evidence that, even in those patients with higher diastolic pressures, there may be less need for prescribing more than one antihypertensive agent and that the doses of prescribed antihypertensive drugs would be significantly less.

These nonpharmacologic concepts were well-accepted, not only by prescribing physicians but also by the general public. Indeed, the benefit proved to be so remarkable that contemporaneously with the publication of the Joint National Committee's Fifth Report (JNC-V), a prevention document indicated that a significant reduction in the number of patients with hypertension in the United States had been achieved. These preliminary findings from the National Health and Nutrition Evaluation Study (NHANES-III) were explained on the widespread acceptance of these lifestyle modification measures. These data, therefore, provided the first evidence that the primary prevention of essential hypertension is a definite possibility. The following are the current lifestyle modification measures that are presently recommended in JNC-V and JNC-VI.

Weight Reduction

Exogenous obesity may, at times, result in erroneous blood pressure measurements in some obese patients with hypertension. However, obesity and hypertension frequently coexist, and a highly significant relationship exists between body weight and blood pressure levels, even in children and adolescents. Weight control not only may result in a reduced arterial pressure in overweight patients with hypertension, but it may permit reduced dosages of antihypertensive drugs in those patients already receiving pharmacotherapy. Thus, weight control is recommended for all overweight hypertensive patients; this is defined by a weight within 15 percent of what is described in life insurance actuarial tables as being "ideal body weight."

More recently, excess body weight has been defined in JNC-VI in terms of a body mass index (body weight in kilograms divided by the height in meters squared) of 27 or greater. This index, although a bit more complicated to calculate, is more closely correlated with the existence of hypertension. In addition, it is now recognized that mid-torso or abdominal obesity (i.e., a waist circumference of $\geq$ 34 inches or $\geq$ 85 cm in women or $\geq$ 39 inches or $\geq$ 98 cm in men) is related to increased cardiovascular morbidity and mortality and an enhanced risk for the development of hypertension, coronary heart disease, dyslipidemias, gout, and diabetes mellitus. A number of studies have shown that reduction in body weight by as little as 10 pounds will be associated with a significant reduction in systolic and diastolic arterial pressure, heart rate, serum cholesterol and uric acid concentrations, and even improved carbohydrate metabolism and management of existing diabetes mellitus. Weight reduction dietary programs are effective, but are commonly fraught with recidivism. It is most important, at this time especially, to express a word of caution with respect to the prescription of pharmacotherapy for a weight reduction program especially in patients with hypertension. Not only will there be risk of potential development of pulmonary hypertension, but systemic arterial hypertension may be precipitated or exacerbated. (For a more detailed discussion of the comorbid condition of obesity and hypertension, the reader is referred to Chapter 10.)

Alcohol Moderation

Excessive alcoholic intake has now been related clearly to elevated arterial pressure. The greater the daily intake of ethanol, the higher the arterial pressure in amounts over one ounce of ethanol consumption per day. Exacerbation of the hypertension may also be attributed to poor adherence to a workable antihypertensive treatment program, long-term control of blood pressure, and subsequent development of "refractory" hypertension. For this reason, moderation of alcohol intake is recommended; this is defined as no more than one ounce of ethanol or its equivalent (i.e., 2 ounces of 100-proof whiskey, 8 ounces of wine, or 24 ounces of beer) daily. JNC-VI cautions further, however, that women absorb more ethanol than men, that lighter weight people are more susceptible than heavier people to the effects of alcohol, and that these groups should be cautioned to limit their daily alcohol intake to no more than 0.5 ounces of ethanol.

Sodium Restriction

As with several other nonpharmacologic treatment modalities, this factor continues to be the subject of much controversy, particularly when it is attributable to all patients with hypertension as well as to the normotensive population of otherwise well individuals. Nevertheless, it is clear that excessive sodium intake does play a critical role in elevating arterial pressure at least in some patients with essential hypertension (estimated by some to range between 35 and 50 percent) and limits the effectiveness of pharmacologic therapy in other patients. A sodium intake of no more than 70 to 100 mEq (2300 mg) per day is a reasonable means to prevent these possibilities. In this respect, it should be kept in mind that almost half of the entire daily sodium intake in most industrialized societies exists in the form of food additives and preservatives of frozen, canned, and processed foods. This includes a seemingly unending alphabetical listing of sodium salts (e.g., acetate, bicarbonate, citrate, fumarate, glutamate, iodide, lactate, malate, nitrite, phosphate, . . .). Furthermore, a sodium restricted diet may obviate antihypertensive drug therapy in patients with high normal or Stage 1 or 2 hypertension and reduce the doses (or number) of prescribed antihypertensive agents. It is also important, in this respect, that the patient who receives diuretic therapy is in a state of secondary hyperaldosteronism and, as such, is more predisposed to the development of hypokalemia with increased dietary sodium intake (since there is more sodium filtered by the glomerulus and available for distal tubular exchange with potassium).

Smoking Cessation

Nicotine raises arterial pressure transiently and is not associated with a persistent increase in blood pressure. While this is true, it is also important to remember that many patients who are "heavy smokers" (more than one, but especially two or more, packages daily) are smoking almost continuously. Hence, this transient elevation in pressure associated in smoking a single cigarette may be considered, more realistically, to be continuous increases of pressure during the waking hours of heavy smokers. It should also be emphasized that long-term cigarette smoking increases the risk of cardiovascular, malignant, and pulmonary diseases and, at least, doubles the risk for the development of coronary heart disease and sudden death. Moreover, these individuals also have a greater chance of developing malignant hypertension and hemorrhagic stroke; cigarette smoking may also interfere with the antihypertensive benefits of certain forms of antihypertensive drug therapy (e.g., propranolol). Thus, the MRC trial in Great Britain and the Mild Hypertension Trial in Australia demonstrated that even though arterial pressure was controlled to the same extent with propranolol as it was with a thiazide diuretic, the β-blocker did not protect the patients taking the drug from myocardial infarction or stroke (as did the diuretic).

Exercise

Although it was previously held that sensible isotonic (e.g., walking, jogging, bicycling, swimming) or aerobic exercise habits are good general health measures and may protect the patient from coronary heart disease, the recent JNC-V and JNC-VI reports present recent evidence that a long-term regular exercise program can control abnormally elevated arterial pressure in some patients with less severe hypertension and adds to a comprehensive antihypertensive program in other patients. This benefit of exercise may be provided not only by virtue of the exercise measures, *per se*, but also by associated weight reduction. In contrast to these isotonic forms of exercise, isometric techniques (e.g., weight-lifting, rowing) may add to the increased total peripheral resistance and afterload imposed on the left ventricle and, thereby, have a negative cardiovascular value (at least in patients with hypertension).

Other Dietary and Nutritional Considerations

There are several new points that have been added to the foregoing lifestyle modification or nonpharmacological treatment recommendations in JNC-VI. The report emphasizes the point that an adequate daily intake of **potassium** is approximately 50 to 90 mmol, which can be obtained from fresh fruits and vegetables (including their juices). Thus, since publication of the prior JNC report an important meta-analysis on the role of dietary potassium intake was reported and indicated that a high dietary potassium intake may be protective against the development of hypertension and may even improve blood pressure control in patients with hypertension. Heretofore, a number of studies dealing with experimental hypertension indicated that, by adding potassium to the diets of animals, arterial pressure will be reduced and cardiovascular damage (including prevention of stroke) may be reversed. Moreover, another important meta-analysis was reported after publication of JNC-V that indicated that when the dose of hydrochlorothiazide (or its equivalent) is reduced from 100 mg down to 25 mg daily, and when potassium wastage is obviated with the coadministration of a potassium-sparing agent, the incidence of sudden cardiac death is reduced. These findings add considerable support to the importance of preventing potassium wastage and of maintaining adequate potassium intake. Of course, it goes without saying that potassium supplementation and pharmacological protection against potassium wastage must be pursued with particular care; this is particularly important in those patients who are taking agents that protect against potassium wastage or with angiotensin converting enzyme inhibitors or angiotensin II (type 1) receptor antagonists.

There is less evidence in support of the need to supplement diets with **calcium** and **magnesium**. It is important to emphasize, however, that a number of reports have indicated that inadequate dietary calcium intake may be associated with a higher prevalence of hypertension. However, studies designed to show that calcium supplementation in the normal diet will reduce blood pressure in patients with hypertension remain unresolved. Similarly, there have been no recommendations to suggest that increased magnesium intake will reduce arterial pressure in patients with hypertension. However, it should also be noted that in those patients with cardiac dysrhythmias secondary to diuretic therapy, significant hypomagnesemia may be associated with hypokalemia; and, in those instances, correction of both deficiencies is indicated to reverse that problem.

It is also important to include in this discussion the well-known frequent concordance of dyslipidemias with hypertensive disease. Thus, one must ascertain the levels of both the high and low density cholesterols as well as the triglyceride levels in all patients with hypertension. More frequently, the careful attention and instruction of patients to follow a prudent diet, low in animal fat, will go far in correction of that problem. There are some reports that a low animal fat diet will reduce arterial pressure; but, at present, although studies have been conducted in normotensive subjects, none has been reported in hypertensive patients.

Stress Reduction

A commonly employed general therapeutic measure is the "glib" instruction to the patient to relax and to avoid emotionally tense situations. Many physicians even prescribe antianxiety agents to help achieve this end. Although relaxation and elimination of tension-related events and activities are desirable for one's overall good health, this is hardly practical and well-founded advice. Furthermore, improvement of extraneous and environmentally produced stressful circumstances will not be associated with remission of hypertensive vascular disease. It is unfortunate that the last seven letters of hypertension is a word that characterizes industrialized societies. Tension should be considered to be related to the increased tone of the arteriolar smooth muscle that is reflected in the increased vascular resistance—the hemodynamic hallmark of hypertensive disease. Studies demonstrate that anxiety-relieving measures—whether drug therapy, psychotherapy, or restructuring of lifestyle—are not associated with adequate control of arterial pressure.

ANNOTATED BIBLIOGRAPHY

The following reports provide detailed data concerning the major early controlled multicenter trials demonstrating safety, efficacy, and reduction of morbidity and mortality by antihypertensive agents.

Veterans Administration Cooperative Study Group on Antihypertension Agents. Effects of treatment on morbidity in hypertension. I. Results in patients with diastolic blood pressure averaging 115 through 129 mm Hg. *JAMA* 1970;202:1028–1034.

Veterans Administration Cooperative Study Group on Antihypertension Agents. Effects of treatment on morbidity in hypertension. II. Results in patients with diastolic blood pressure averaging 90 through 114 mm Hg. *JAMA* 1970;213: 1143–1152.

Veterans Administration Cooperative Study Group on Antihypertension Agents: III. Influence of age, diastolic pressure, and prior cardiovascular disease. Further analysis of side effects. *Circulation* 1972;45;991–1004.

Hypertension Detection and Follow-Up Program Cooperative Group: Five-year findings of the Hypertension Detection and Follow-Up Program: I. Reduction in mortality of persons with high blood pressure, including mild hypertension. *JAMA* 1979;242:2562–2571.

Multiple Risk Factor Intervention Trial Research Group: Multiple Risk Factor Intervention Trial: Risk factor changes and mortality results. *JAMA* 1982;248:1465–1477.

European Working Party on High Blood Pressure in the Elderly: Mortality and morbidity results from the European Working Party on High Blood Pressure in the Elderly. *Lancet* 1985;1:1349–1354.

Management Committee: The Australian therapeutic trial in mild hypertension. *Lancet* 1980;I:1261–1267.

The following reports provided the first and soundest meta-analysis of the first 14 multicenter antihypertensive drug trials that demonstrated reduction of morbidity and mortality by the diuretics and beta-adrenergic receptor blocking drugs from stroke and coronary heart disease. The following references similarly demonstrated similar findings in elderly patients with hypertension.

MacMahon S, Peto R, Cutler J, et al: Blood pressure stroke and coronary heart disease. I. Prolonged differences in blood pressure: Prospective observational studies corrected for the regression dilution bias. *Lancet* 1990;335:765–774.

Thijs L, Fagard R, Lijnen P, Staessen J, Van Hoot R, Amery A: A meta-analysis of outcome trials in elderly hypertensives. *J Hypertens* 1992;10:1103–1109.

The following three papers demonstrated reduction of morbidity and mortality from stroke and coronary heart disease in elderly patients with isolated systolic hypertension using diuretics and beta-adrenergic receptor blocking drugs.

SHEP Cooperative Research Group: Prevention of stroke by antihypertensive drug treatment in older persons with isolated systolic hypertension: Final results of the Systolic Hypertension in the Elderly Program (SHEP). *JAMA* 1991;265: 3255–3264.

MRC Working Party. Medical Research Council trail of treatment of hypertension in older adults: principal results. *BMJ* 1992;304:405–412.

Dahlöf B, Lindholm LH, Hansson L, Schersten B, Ekhom T, Wester PO: Morbidity and mortality in the Swedish Trial in Old Patients with Hypertension (STOP-Hypertension). *Lancet* 1991;338:1281–1285.

The following two reports demonstrated the hemodynamic mechanisms of weight reduction in hypertensive patients with exogenous obesity and reviews the pathophysiology of obesity of hypertension respectively.

Reisin E, Frohlich ED, Messerli FH, Dreslinski GR, Dunn FG, Jones MM, Batson HM Jr: Cardiovascular changes after weight reduction in obesity hypertension. *Ann Intern Med* 1983;98:315–319.

Reisin E, Frohlich ED: Effects of weight reduction on arterial pressure. *J Chronic Dis* 1982;35:887–891.

The following reports present the epidemiological and clinical evidence supporting nonpharmacological modalities in reducing blood pressure and controlling hypertension.

Frohlich ED, Gifford R Jr, Horan M, Kaplan NM, Maxwell MH, Payne G, Roccella EJ, Shapiro AP, Weiss S, Bowler AE: Nonpharmacologic approaches to the control of high blood pressure. Report of the Subcommittee on Nonpharmacologic Therapy of the Joint National Committee on Detection, Evaluation, and Treatment of High Blood Pressure, 1984. *Hypertension* 1986;8:444–467.

Frohlich, ED: Multicenter clinical trials: Potential influence of consumer education. *Hypertension* 1987;9(III):75–79.

The Joint National Committee on the Detection, Evaluation, and Treatment of High Blood Pressure: The 1984 Report of the Joint National Committee on Detection, Evaluation, and Treatment of High Blood Pressure. *Arch Intern Med* 1984;144:1045–1057.

Joint National Committee on the Detection, Evaluation, and Treatment of Blood Pressure (member): The 1992 Report of the Joint National Committee on the Detection, Evaluation, and Treatment of Blood Pressure (JNC-V). *Arch Intern Med* 1993;153:154–183.

Joint National Committee on the Detection, Evaluation, and Treatment of Blood Pressure: The Sixth Report of the Joint National Committee on the Detection, Evaluation, and Treatment of Blood Pressure. *Arch Intern Med* 1997;157:2413–2446.

National High Blood Pressure Education Program, Working Group Report on Primary Prevention of Hypertension. *Arch Intern Med* 1993;153:186–208.

Wassertheil-Smoller S, Blaufox MD, Oberman AS, Langford HG, Davis BR, Wylie-Rosett J. The Trial of Antihypertensive Interventions and Management (TAIM) Study: Adequate weight loss, alone and combined with drug therapy in the treatment of mild hypertension. *Arch Intern Med* 1992;152:131–136.

Stamler R, Stamler J, Grimm R, et al: Nutritional therapy for high blood pressure: Final report of a four-year randomized controlled tria—the Hypertension Control Program. *JAMA* 1987;257:1484–1491.

Intersalt Cooperative Research Group: Intersalt: An international study of electrolyte excretion and blood pressure. Result for 24 hour urinary sodium and potassium excretion. *BMJ* 1988;297:319–328.

Blair SN, Kohl HW III, Paffenbarger RS Jr, Clark DG, Cooper KH, Gibbons LW: Physical fitness and all-cause mortality: A prospective study of healthy men and women. *JAMA* 1989;262:2395–2401.

The following chapter from Hurst's therapeutic textbook presents further evidence of lifestyle modifications and nondrug effects in controlling elevated arterial pressure.

Frohlich ED: Hypertension: Essential. In: *Current Therapy in Cardiovascular Disease*, 4th ed. (Hurst JW, ed). Mosby–Year Book, Philadelphia, 1994, pp. 291–299.

The following very recent meta-analysis strongly suggests a hypotensive action for dietary potassium supplement action—especially for those patients who need to reduce sodium intake.

Whelton PK, He J, Cutler JA, Brancati PL, Appel LJ, Follmann D, Klag MJ: The effects of oral potassium on blood pressure: A quantitative overview of randomized, controlled clinical trials. *JAMA* 1997 277:1624–1632.

Chapter 4

Clinical Pharmacology of Antihypertensive Agents

In this chapter we shall discuss each of the presently available classes of antihypertensive agents in some detail. In the following sections we shall discuss individualized approaches for specifically identified specialized groups of patients or those with specific complications from hypertension. For the purpose of brevity, however, the reader is referred to the "suggested references" sections of this book and other various review publications primarily by the author that provide detailed references for specific statements made concerning the various antihypertensive drugs, their mechanisms of action, hemodynamic effects, and their clinical effects and potential adverse experiences.

DIURETICS

This group of antihypertensive drugs has been available for almost 40 years, and they continue to remain the mainstay of antihypertensive therapy. Inherent in their use are the concept and rationale for low-sodium diet therapy for reversing severe hypertensive disease and for enhancing the effectiveness of other antihypertensive drugs. To be effective as the sole therapy, however, dietary sodium restriction usually must be less than 200 mg/day. One must remember that approximately one-half of dietary sodium is provided by salt; the other half is found in food additives and preservatives. Since this form of diet therapy is highly impractical, we frequently rely upon oral natriuretic agents. There are three classes of oral diuretic agents: thiazides and their congeners, "loop" diuretics, and potassium-retaining agents.

Thiazide Congeners

These agents, including chlorothiazide, hydrochlorothiazide, and a long list of their chemical congeners, are all quite similar in action, side effects, and dosages. One tablet of any one agent is generally equivalent to another compound in its antihypertensive and natriuretic potency, as well as in its hypokalemic potential for other side effects. According to the most recent Joint National Committee's (JNC) recommendations of the fifth and sixth reports (i.e., JNC-V and JNC-VI), the thiazide diuretics (and their congeners), in contrast to the "loop" diuretics, should be considered first among the classes of antihypertensive agents selected for initial therapy of patients with uncomplicated, essential hypertension. The thiazides are the preferable diuretic agents unless the patients had previously demonstrated intolerance or idiosyncracy to these compounds or unless renal excretory function of the hypertensive patient is abnormal. With increasing diuretic dosages (up to 500 or 1000 mg of chlorothiazide or 50 or 100 mg of hydrochlorothiazide), there will be increasing diuretic and associated metabolic effects; larger doses offer little more natriuretic and diuretic efficacy but may enhance the development of their inherent metabolic side effects (e.g., hypokalemia, hyperuricemia). On the other hand, if the patient has impaired renal excretory function, a loop diuretic may be prescribed in doses that may be progressively increased until, eventually, adequate diuresis is achieved.

It is important to recognize that the thiazides were originally prescribed in doses equivalent to 100 mg hydrochlorothiazide (or more). This explains the greater likelihood for development of metabolic side effects (i.e., hypokalemia, hyperuricemia, carbohydrate intolerance, possible hyperlipidemia, and modestly elevated serum creatinine) and their associated effects. However, with use of the more recent JNC (III through VI) recommendations of 12.5 to 25 mg initial dosing of hydrochlorothiazide, and to 50 mg in full dose, these adverse side effects and clinical consequences have been less pronounced.

The thiazides reduce arterial pressure initially primarily as a result of a contracted extracellular (plasma and interstitial) fluid volume and, later, as a consequence of reduced total peripheral resistance. Thus, initially, following its administration, there is an immediate decrease in plasma volume and cardiac output that is associated with a reduction in total body sodium and water. Then, within a few days, arterial pressure falls (by approximately 10 to 15 percent), associated with further natriuresis and diuresis. After about six weeks, the plasma volume and cardiac output return toward pretreatment levels, and the reduced arterial pressure is then associated with a decreased total peripheral resistance. The precise mechanism for this decreased arteriolar resistance is still poorly understood, but current thinking relates to local generation of prostacyclines or other vasodilators through autocrine/paracrine mechanisms.

In addition to its hypotensive effect, there is an additional consequence of volume contraction: an attenuated response to pressor agents and enhanced responsiveness to depressor substances. This mechanism provides an explanation for antihypertensive synergism of the diuretics with other antihypertensive drugs (e.g., vasodilators, β-blockers, antiadrenergic compounds, angiotensin converting enzyme inhibitors). Other mechanisms that have been offered to explain the antihypertensive action of diuretics include: altered transmembrane ionic potential across the vascular smooth muscle cell membrane; altered responsiveness to endogenously generated neural stimuli and norepinephrine release; reduced "waterlogging" of the hypertensive arteriolar wall; and, as already suggested, through autocrine/paracrine mechanisms that induce local vasodilators. More than likely, no one mechanism is totally operative, and all (or, possibly, even others) may participate in their overall antihypertensive action.

The thiazide diuretics promote natriuresis through inhibition of carbonic anhydrase and of active sodium reabsorption in the proximal and distal tubules. With natriuresis and volume contraction, the kidney releases renin from the juxtaglomerular apparatus, leading to the secondary generation of angiotensin II and consequent adrenal cortical release of aldosterone, thereby providing a positive feedback to the natriuretic stimulus. In addition, potassium and chloride ions are also lost in the urine, thereby inducing hypokalemic alkalosis with an alkaline urine (i.e., secondary hyperaldosteronism) that may be confused with other causes of hypokalemic alkalosis from hyperaldosteronism (e.g., renal arterial disease, primary aldosteronism, cardiac failure). Most important, with excessive dietary sodium intake, this secondary hyperaldosteronism can exacerbate the hypokalemic effect of the diuretic by favoring sodium-for-potassium exchange at the distal tubule. Hence, one important means of reducing the hypokalemia produced by thiazides is to restrict daily sodium intake.

The thiazides also increase tubular reabsorption of urate and increase plasma uric acid concentration. If this is severe enough, symptomatic gout may result. Therefore, if the uric acid level is borderline or elevated at the outset of therapy or if there is a personal or family history of gout, it should be rechecked intermittently during treatment in anticipation of the potential problem of gout. Should hyperuricemic levels approach 10.0 to 11.0 mg per 100 ml (or more), specific drug therapy may be prescribed to reduce serum uric acid concentration. This may be achieved with the uricosuric agent probenecid or with allopurinol, an inhibitor of the enzyme xanthine oxidase that reduces uric acid synthesis. Alternatively, other antihypertensive agents that are also effective for initial antihypertensive therapy may be substituted instead of the diuretic.

The thiazides may also induce carbohydrate intolerance or hyperglycemia of varying degrees. For the most part, much of the metabolic side effect problems may depend upon the dose used of the thiazide. In any event, when more recent dose recommendations of thiazides are followed, the risk of development of diabetes with hypoglycemic therapy is not any greater than that for any other antihypertensive therapeutic class. One mechanism underlying carbohydrate intolerance has been explained by the ability of the diuretic to inhibit insulin release from the beta cells of the pancreatic islets. Another factor that may participate in this "diabetogenic" state is the hypokalemic milieu engendered by the diuretic, but this concept remains unresolved. Still another aspect to this controversy is the possible state of "end-organ" hyporesponsiveness or insensitivity to insulin in patients with essential hypertension as well as with obesity, diabetes mellitus, and hyperlipidemia; this may also become exacerbated by these diuretic agents. In my experience, however, overt insulin-dependent diabetes mellitus will not result *de novo* in hypertensive patients who do not already have abnormal carbohydrate tolerance prior to initiation of the diuretic. Should clinical diabetes mellitus develop, this does not necessarily require discontinuance of the thiazide, and it may be possible to prevent expression of the clinical problem with a lower dose of the diuretic (12.5 to 50 mg hydrochlorothiazide) or by controlling the overall problem with either dietotherapy and weight reduction alone, an oral hypoglycemic agent, or, if necessary, insulin. Alternatively, as already indicated, should this problem be of sufficient clinical concern, another agent from a different class of antihypertensive drugs may be substituted for the initial diuretic therapy of hypertension.

The problem of hypokalemia had been minimized clinically in the earlier years of thiazide therapy, especially in the United States. But, as suggested, we have learned relatively recently that lower doses of the thiazides provide similar control of arterial pressure with less severe hypokalemia and other metabolic side effects. Furthermore, as already indicated, reduced dietary sodium intake (in the background of diuretic-induced secondary hyperaldosteronism) minimizes the hypokalemic effect of the sodium-for-potassium exchange mechanism at the distal tubule. Addition of spironolactone or amiloride will augment the hypotensive effect of the thiazide; but, in contrast, triamterene does not. However, all three of these potassium-sparing agents protect against hypokalemia. Symptoms of hypokalemia include polyuria, nocturia, muscle weakness, and atrial or ventricular ectopic activity. These symptoms should be corrected with supplemental potassium or the addition of a potassium-retaining agent. If primary hyperaldosteronism is considered a feature of this problem, the diuretic should be discontinued pending further clinical evaluation; and, once the diagnosis is established, the disease should be treated more specifically. If the patient is receiving digitalis or there are other explanations for aggravating the hypokalemia (e.g., laxative abuse, chronic diarrhea, vomiting, or an intestinal villous adenoma), reduced serum potassium levels should be corrected or an alternative antihypertensive agent should be considered. Angiotensin-converting enzyme (ACE) inhibitors should be used with extreme caution (if at all) in patients receiving potassium supplementation or any of the potassium-retaining agents, as well as in patients with severely impaired renal excretory function.

Other side effects that have been related to the thiazides include hyperlipidemia, occasional maculopapular rashes, reduction in the circulating number of any or all of the blood-formed elements, hypercalcemia, and transient reduction in renal excretory function as a consequence of reduced renal blood flow. The latter may be more apparent in patients with preexisting impaired renal excretory function. Under those circumstances, use of a diuretic should not be a deterrent from persistence of antihypertensive therapy; should therapy be relaxed, the long-term consequences may be even more disastrous.

In this regard, one should consider therapeutic alternatives to diuretics. Although not diuretic agents, the calcium antagonists exert a natriuretic action that may be most useful for those patients who might have been considered to receive diuretics. These patients may be among the elderly and black population, or they may be among those patients with parenchymal renal disease, steroid-dependent hypertensions, or angina pectoris unable to take beta-blocking drugs. Although the issue of diuretic-induced hyperlipidemia continues to remain highly controversial, many authorities (perhaps the majority) believe that the elevated lipid level that may be produced in some patients will return to pretreatment levels with time (i.e., usually within a year). It is my feeling that if hyperlipidemia is present prior to initiating treatment or if it is induced by the diuretic, other therapeutic options are available and may be equally efficacious.

The thiazide diuretics, as indicated, are considered "preferred" for initial treatment of patients with hypertension because they have demonstrated (along with the beta blockers) reduced morbidity and mortality in controlled multicenter trials. Among those patients who are more likely to respond to initial monotherapy are (a) those who are volume-dependent and have lower pretreatment plasma renin activity, (b) those who have a history of renal parenchymal infections (even if present renal excretory function is normal), (c) those who have essential hypertension with lower plasma renin activity (e.g., blacks, obese individuals), (d) those who have steroid-dependent forms of hypertension (e.g., primary aldosteronism, Cushing's disease or syndrome, and perhaps oral-contraceptive-induced hypertension, caused by taking exogenous steroidal agents), and (e) elderly hypertensives with diastolic as well as isolated systolic hypertension.

Loop Diuretics

Bumetanide, ethacrynic acid, and furosemide are the most potent diuretic agents in clinical use. Unlike the thiazides, these agents exert their natriuretic action by inhibiting sodium transport at the ascending limb of the loop of Henle. Since more of the filtered sodium is delivered to the distal tubule for exchange, a greater degree of potassium wastage will result. The onset of action of these agents is more immediate and abrupt, with diuresis frequently noted within 20 minutes of the oral dose. As a result, the diuresis is more rapid and evident than with the thiazides and their congeners, the rebound retention of sodium and water may be more pronounced, and there may be a greater degree of potassium wastage. For the foregoing reasons, these compounds should be reserved for the following patients: those who cannot take the thiazides; those in whom a more prompt diuresis is desired; those with renal functional impairment; or those for whom an intravenous diuretic is clinically necessary. In those patients with renal functional impairment, unlike the thiazides, the dose–response curve of the loop agents is linear. For example, if an effect is not achieved with a daily furosemide dosage of 40 or 80 mg, it may be increased (e.g., 160 mg or more) until diuresis is achieved. Indeed, some nephrologists have reported that diuresis may eventually be achieved with doses of 2000 mg.

Thus, the "loop diuretics" are not recommended for patients with uncomplicated, essential hypertension unless a significant degree of impaired renal function or thiazide intolerance exists. And, in patients with secondary hyperaldosteronism (e.g., congestive heart failure), particular care should be exercised to prevent hypokalemia and cardiac dysrhythmias and a very real potential sudden cardiac death. One final important, but occasionally overlooked, indication for these agents is in hypertensive patients who are already receiving antihypertensive drugs, including the maximum daily doses of a thiazide. These patients may have developed pseudotolerance as a consequence of intravascular volume expansion, and it may be overcome by switching to the more potent loop-acting agent. The net effect of this therapeutic maneuver is to promote a more vigorous depletion of retained sodium and water. Once this effect is achieved, the overall treatment program might be restructured to obviate multiple diuretic usage.

Potassium-Sparing Agents

Spironolactone   This diuretic is discussed separately because it promotes diuresis through a very specific mechanism, namely, distal tubular inhibition of the action of aldosterone. Thus, by interfering with the aldosterone-mediated sodium-for-potassium ion exchange mechanism, natriuresis and diuresis are effected without wastage of the potassium ion. Since much of the obligate sodium ion transport occurs at the level of the proximal tubule, the potency of spironolactone is not as great as that of thiazides. Nevertheless, spironolactone is particularly useful, either alone or in combination with a thiazide compound, for patients with primary and secondary hyperaldosteronism. Its antihypertensive effect, however, is not markedly different from the thiazides in these patients, but protection of total body potassium can be provided. Hence, in patients with hyperaldosteronism, the major value of spironolactone is that it achieves a significant sodium and water excretion without depleting potassium (even when used in combination with a thiazide). Because spironolactone is effective in secondary hyperaldosteronism states, it may be of particular value in patients receiving digitalis (with cardiac failure) to correct or prevent that degree of hypokalemia which may predispose the patient to cardiac dysrhythmias. Since spironolactone resembles progesterone in its chemical configuration, its side effects may include gynecomastia and mastodynia, a complaint not infrequently reported particularly in men. Sometimes this problem may be alleviated by dose reduction rather than by totally withdrawing the drug. The physician should also be aware of the potential for the development of hyperkalemia in patients with impaired renal function or if the patient is also taking an angiotensin-converting enzyme (ACE) inhibitor. This should be of special importance in patients with chronic renal diseases or with cardiac failure; in these people, supplemental potassium with or without a potassium-sparing agent, should be used with extreme caution.

Amiloride and Triamterene   These two agents are structurally related and act on the same non-aldosterone-dependent active sodium-for-potassium renal tubular transport mechanism. Therefore, their action is entirely different from spironolactone. Both agents reduce arterial pressure when used with a thiazide to preserve potassium. However, although triamterene has an amiloride-like potassium-sparing action, it has minimal, if any, diuretic and antihypertensive properties. Moreover, as emphasized with spironolactone, these agents should be used with caution in patients with impaired renal function and, probably not at all, in patients receiving ACE inhibitors because of the potential of severe hyperkalemia.

BETA-ADRENERGIC BLOCKING AGENTS

The beta-adrenergic blocking drugs have been considered as alternative agents for the initial treatment of hypertension for many years. As already indicated, these two classes of antihypertensive agents are the only ones that have demonstrated reduction of cardiovascular morbidity and mortality in controlled multicenter trials. These agents inhibit stimulation of cardiovascular beta-adrenergic receptor sites by adrenergic neurohumoral substances (i.e., norepinephrine, epinephrine) that are released from the nerve ending or adrenal medulla. By inhibiting beta-receptor stimulation, the effects of peripheral arteriolar dilation (beta$_2$-receptor-mediated) and of increased heart rate, myocardial contractility, and myocardial metabolism are minimized. Moreover, because beta-adrenergic receptor sites in the kidney are also inhibited, renal renin release is inhibited. The result is a decreased arterial pressure that is associated with a reduced cardiac output, although (the calculated) total peripheral resistance increases. Heart rate and myocardial contractility is also inhibited. The reduced cardiac output (often by 20 to 25 percent) may not be associated with proportionate reductions in all organ blood flows. Renal blood flow and excretory function may not be diminished at all with beta-blocking therapy since reduction in organ blood flows depends upon the number and affinity of beta-adrenergic receptor sites in each of the respective organ circulation. Thus, even though arterial pressure reduction is associated with reduced cardiac output and increased total peripheral resistance, effects on the heart and kidney may not be as detrimental as first conceived. Actually, myocardial oxygen demand is reduced and renal blood flow may be unchanged or increased as renal vascular resistance diminishes. By contrast, blood flow to the skeletal muscles and splanchnic organs is indeed reduced. The reduction in skeletal muscle blood flow may explain the fatigue experienced on exercise by some patients. Another important feature of these agents is the lack of expansion of intravascular volume as arterial pressure declines. Nevertheless, diuretics clearly augment the antihypertensive effectiveness of the beta-blocking drugs, and they are frequently prescribed in combination.

At present, 14 beta-blocking agents are available for antihypertensive therapy; carvedilol and labetalol possess in a single molecule both alpha- and beta-adrenergic receptor inhibiting properties. Four agents (acebutolol, betaxolol, bisoprolol, carteolol, penbutolol, and pindolol) possess cardiostimulatory (intrinsic sympathomimetic activity) properties. Hence, they may not reduce heart rate and cardiac output as much as other agents. They may, therefore, be of some value in patients with preexisting bradycardia or low cardiac output syndromes. The so-called cardioselective beta$_1$ blockers (acebutolol, atenolol, metoprolol) probably exceed the property of cardioselectivity in the doses prescribed for the treatment of hypertension and angina pectoris. Nevertheless, they may have been of some value to patients who live in those climates and who have symptoms of Raynaud's phenomenon or peripheral arterial insufficiency in winter months. Among the non-cardioselective agents are nadolol and timolol.

Because of the foregoing physiologic and pharmacologic actions, these agents have been found to be of particular value for the initial treatment of certain patients with hypertension. This includes patients with hyperdynamic circulatory states and who exhibit faster heart rates, symptoms of cardiac awareness, and palpitations related to enhanced cardiac contractility, and extrasystoles may be more responsive to beta blockers. White patients may respond better to beta-blocker monotherapy than black patients; however, when the agent is combined with a diuretic, the efficacy is similar between the two racial groups.

Since beta-blocking therapy is also effective for a number of other clinical conditions, it may be wise to utilize this therapy for the initial treatment of hypertension in those patients. These circumstances may include patients with hyperdynamic beta-adrenergic circulatory state or hyperkinetic heart syndrome, patients with angina pectoris or a previous history of myocardial infarction, patients with cardiac dysrhythmias responsive to beta blockers (such as catecholamine-induced), patients with idiopathic mitral valvular prolapse syndrome, patients with migraine headaches, patients with skeletal muscle tremors, and patients with glaucoma (who may already receive beta-blocker eye drops without having systemic side effects). Because of the systemic inhibition of beta receptors, this form of initial antihypertensive therapy should not be used in patients with a history of asthma, chronic obstructive lung disease, heart block of second degree or more, or severe peripheral arterial insufficiency. In recent years, beta blockers have been used in patients with cardiac failure, but particular care concerning exacerbating this problem should be made, particularly early in this difficult treatment effort. Notwithstanding this cautionary note, some new beta-blocking compounds with beta-1 receptor vasodilator agonism and beta-2 cardiac muscle antagonism have been approved (e.g., carvedilol) for treatment of specific patients with cardiac failure, and the preliminary results look good. Still another beta-blocker (sotalol) is useful for certain cardiac dysrhythmias.

If full doses of the selected beta-blocking agent do not control arterial pressure, the addition of a diuretic or even a calcium antagonist may be effective, particularly in the patient with coronary artery disease. However, caution should be exercised in the latter circumstance, since the negative and chronotropic effects of some calcium antagonists may exacerbate that same effect already provided by the beta-blocking agent. Finally, if side effects such as fatigue, depression, hallucination, or nightmares preclude further use of the chosen beta blocker, it might be worthwhile to select an alternative beta-blocking drug before switching to another class of antihypertensive agents.

ADRENERGIC INHIBITING COMPOUNDS

With the present array of sympatholytic compounds available, it is now possible for the clinician to dissect pharmacologically the autonomic nervous system. The first drugs introduced were the ganglion-blocking drugs; agents that selectively inhibit sympathetic nervous activity (in the brain or at the postganglionic neuronal terminal) were introduced later. Among the latter agents were those that depleted the neurohumoral (norepinephrine) agents from postganglionic nerve endings and the central nervous system. The centrally acting agents that stimulate alpha-adrenergic receptors in cardiovascular medullary centers (e.g., nucleus tractus solitarius) that reduce adrenergic outflow to the cardiovascular system and kidney were introduced still later.

Ganglion Blockers

The ganglion-blocking agents reduce arterial pressure by diminishing autonomic outflow to the heart and vascular smooth muscle at the level of thoracodorsal autonomic ganglia. The net effect is a reduction in arteriolar and venular smooth muscle tone that results in vasodilation. The venodilation promotes peripheral pooling of blood and diminishes venous return to the heart, an effect that is enhanced in the upright posture with dependent venous blood pooling. Arteriolar dilation decreases total peripheral and organ vascular resistances. Autonomic inhibition of the heart results in the attenuation of cardiac reflexes. Thus, with upright posture, hypotension results from reduced venous return to the heart, attenuation of normal reflexive increases in heart rate and myocardial contractility. Other examples of inhibited compensatory reflexes are shown by the abolition of the overshoot phase of the Valsalva maneuver, augmentation of postural hypotension and the "tilt-back" overshoot of arterial pressure when the patient returns to the supine position or is in postexercise hypotension. The former phenomenon is explained on the basis of the sudden return of pooled blood to the circulation, and the latter is explained on the basis of redistribution of circulating blood into the vasodilated skeletal musculature when the patient remains upright. These same hemodynamic effects obtained with the ganglion blockers may also be observed after administration of postganglionic inhibitors (e.g., guanethidine) that deplete the sympathetic nerve endings of norepinephrine; however, in this situation one does not observe the inhibition of parasympathetic function which is also observed with the ganglion blockers.

Although the ganglion blockers had been the mainstay of treatment for severe hypertension a number of years ago, these agents are now used almost exclusively in the intravenous formulation for the immediate and controlled treatment of certain severe hypertensive emergencies or for control of arterial pressure during certain operative (e.g., neurosurgical) procedures. In these circumstances, trimethaphan camsylate is infused intravenously (1 mg/ml) to produce instantaneous control of arterial pressure; pressure will rise promptly with reduction (or cessation) of its infusion. Antihypertensive effectiveness is enhanced by upright posture (i.e., elevating the head of the bed) with the concomitant use of diuretics or with blood loss.

With this and all other adrenergic inhibiting as well as the direct-acting smooth muscle vasodilating agents, the phenomenon of pseudotolerance (intravascular volume expansion after control of pressure is achieved) will frequently occur unless a diuretic is administered simultaneously. This explains why their hypotensive action is enhanced by diuretics. The ganglion-blocking drugs also inhibit parasympathetic nerve activity; as a consequence, intestinal and urinary bladder smooth muscle activity is also inhibited, thereby predisposing the patient to severe paralytic ileus and urinary retention. An additional side effect (not usually a complaint during intravenous infusion) is loss of penile erectile function.

Rauwolfia Alkaloids

Included in this group are a number of agents having varying potencies and abilities to deplete neuronal tissue (brain, adrenal, and postganglionic sympathetic nerve endings) of the biogenic amines. These compounds had been used with greater frequency in the earlier years of antihypertensive drug therapy; they are still used widely around the world. When administered by injection (e.g., reserpine, 1.0 to 5.0 mg), they have been effective in treating hypertensive emergencies and thyrotoxicosis. A test injection of 0.25 or 0.5 mg is worthwhile to administer in order to avoid excessive pressure reduction with larger doses. In recent years, with the introduction of newer agents having less bothersome side effects (e.g., reserpine-induced obtunded sensorium or depression), they have been used rarely for hypertensive emergencies. However, when administered orally, they serve as mild antihypertensive compounds; but they must be used with a diuretic since when they are used alone, their antihypertensive effect is minimal. They reduce arterial pressure through a fall in total peripheral resistance associated with a decreased heart rate and an unchanged cardiac output. One bothersome side effect is nasal stuffiness relating to the vasodilating action. Other important side effects include postural hypotension, bradycardia, overriding parasympathetic gastrointestinal tract stimulation, mental depression, and sexual dysfunction. The mental depression may be most subtle and should be considered when evaluating any patient who has been receiving these agents over a prolonged time, particularly if there is any concern about behavioral changes. The reports of associated increased prevalence of breast carcinoma were subsequently found to be unsubstantiated, and concern of this problem is unfounded.

Postganglionic Neuronal Depletors

Included among this class of drugs are guanethidine and guanadrel. The former compound has been available for patients with more severe hypertension for about 35 years. The latter was introduced more recently for patients with less severe hypertension. Both compounds have similar pharmacologic actions, although in the relatively lower doses offered with guanadrel, the side effects are less bothersome. Guanethidine has a prolonged delay (up to 48 or 72 hours) in its onset of hypotensive action, which, once achieved, may persist for days or weeks (even as much as one month) after the drug has been discontinued. Both agents demonstrate hemodynamic effects similar to those of the ganglion-blocking drugs, although the additional effects of parasympathetic inhibition of neural function is absent. There is a fall in arteriolar resistance, peripheral venodilation, decreased venous return to the heart with a consequent decrease in cardiac output, and attenuated cardiovascular reflexive adjustments; the associated reduced renal blood flow may impair renal excretory function. In the patient with adequate pretreatment renal functional reserve, the decrease in function observed with treatment may readjust itself—albeit, perhaps, less completely—in patients with already compromised renal function. Additional side effects include bradycardia, orthostatic hypotension, increased frequency of bowel movements and diarrhea (from unopposed parasympathetic function), and retrograde ejaculation.

These adrenolytic compounds are taken up by the postganglionic nerve endings, thereby inhibiting norepinephrine reuptake. As a result, the postganglionic nerve endings become depleted of the neurohumoral substance. This concept is important since the commonly used tricyclic antidepressant drugs (e.g., imipramine [Tofranil], desipramine [Pertofrane], amitriptyline [Elavil], protriptyline [Vivactil]) inhibit the nerve-ending ability to incorporate guanethidine and guanadrel. Thus, these tricyclic antidepressants antagonize the antihypertensive actions of these potent antihypertensive drugs; and, conversely, when the antidepressant drug is discontinued, arterial pressure may fall suddenly and precipitously.

Centrally Acting Postsynaptic Alpha-Adrenergic Agonists

Methyldopa still continues to be a widely used agent worldwide for over 35 years. Although originally thought to reduce arterial pressure through an inhibition of the enzyme dopa-decarboxylase, it was later postulated to work by false neural transmission. This action implies conversion of the drug alpha-methyldopa to its less biologically active amine alpha-methylnorepinephrine, which, in turn, binds to peripheral alpha-adrenergic receptor sites in competition with the norepinephrine. More recently, however, its antihypertensive action has been shown to be mediated through its false neurohumoral substance, alpha-methylnorepinephrine, in the brain. The false neurotransmitter stimulates postsynaptic alpha receptor sites in the brain (i.e., nucleus tractus solitarii), thereby resulting in reduced adrenergic outflow from the medullary centers to the cardiovascular system and kidney, resulting in decreased arterial pressure. This is achieved hemodynamically through a fall in arteriolar resistance and a lesser fall in venous tone than observed with the above-described agents. Consequently, cardiac output and renal blood flow are not reduced as much; therefore, postural hypotension is less commonly observed with these agents.

The most common side effects include dry mouth, lethargy, easy fatigability, somnolence, and sexual dysfunction. These complaints may be attributed to methyldopa's central action and may disappear shortly after therapy is discontinued. Other less common side effects include Coombs' test-positive reactions (much less frequently, hemolytic anemia), high fever after initial drug doses, and hepatotoxicity, all of which remit upon withdrawal of therapy.

Clonidine, guanabenz, and guanfacine, although chemically different from methyldopa, share certain pharmacologic actions with that agent. These agents also have little direct peripheral arteriolar dilating properties, and they reduce arterial pressure primarily through a decreased vascular resistance as a result of central stimulation of the postsynaptic alpha-adrenergic receptor sites in the nuclei tractii solitarii. The result is reduced adrenergic outflow from the brain that also inhibits renal renin production.

A word is indicated concerning the **clonidine suppression test**. Occasionally, when the possibility of pheochromocytoma is entertained as a secondary cause of hypertension, the differential diagnosis may be difficult. The patient may have complaints that are suggestive of the adrenal catecholamine-producing tumor and measurement of circulating catecholamine levels is indicated. The normal blood level of norepinephrine is usually less than 100 ng/ml; and levels in patients with the adrenal medullary tumor are usually in excess of 600 ng/ml. Since catecholamine levels resulting from a pheochromocytoma are not usually suppressible, and there may be some question in those patients with intermediary levels (between 100 and 600 ng/ml), this suppression test may be of value. Clonidine is administered in three successive hourly doses of 0.1 mg, and the pretest elevated catecholamine level is reduced to normal levels in patients who do not have the adrenal tumor. Patients with essential hypertension and borderline elevated levels of norepinephrine and patients with idiopathic mitral valve prolapse will demonstrate a suppression of the elevated levels.

These agents share many of the side effects of other adrenergic inhibiting compounds as described above. One particular side effect which seems to be more commonly associated with clonidine is the possibility of a precipitous rebound of arterial pressure after its abrupt withdrawal. When this does occur, symptoms of palpitations and tachycardia can be treated with a beta-adrenergic blocking drug, and the pressor phenomenon may be counteracted with the injection of an alpha-adrenergic blocking drug (e.g., phentolamine) and/or reinstitution of the clonidine or another adrenergic inhibitor or another antihypertensive agent. In recent years, clonidine has been made available as a transdermal patch (long-acting) medication that apparently has made these rebound episodes less likely. As with the other adrenergic inhibitors, when used alone they are usually associated with intravascular volume expansion and pseudotolerance. Hence, they are not generally considered among the initial therapeutic options for the treatment of hypertension.

Pre- and Postsynaptic (Alpha-1- and Alpha-2-Receptor Antagonists)

The alpha-1- and alpha-2- receptor blocking drugs (e.g., dibenzylene) developed earlier have very limited usefulness for the treatment of most ambulatory hypertensive patients. They continue to be used (e.g., phentolamine, 5 to 10 mg intravenously) for unexplained pressor episodes that suggest excessive release of catecholamines. Thus, they may be used by continuous intravenous infusion for the patient with a pheochromocytoma crisis or in a patient with pressor crisis-associated clonidine withdrawal. Since pargyline hydrochloride and other monoamine oxidase inhibitors are still marketed as antihypertensive and, more frequently, as antidepressant agents, they also may be associated with hypertensive crisis after ingestion of certain foodstuffs (e.g., Chianti wine, marinated foods, certain cheeses) containing tyramine. The alpha-adrenergic blocking compounds are valuable in treating these pressor crisis episodes because the tyramine contained in the food releases stored norepinephrine from the nerve endings, and the released neurohumoral substance is less able to be degraded in the presence of monoamine oxidase inhibitors.

Postsynaptic (Peripheral) Alpha$_1$ Antagonists

There are two types of alpha-adrenergic receptors in the periphery. When the postsynaptic alpha$_1$ receptors are stimulated by the catecholamines released from the postganglionic nerve ending, arteriolar and venular constriction occur. When presynaptic alpha$_2$ receptors are stimulated, further release of the norepinephrine from the nerve ending into the synoptic cleft is inhibited. Thus, in contradistinction to the alpha$_1$- and alpha$_2$-receptor-inhibiting compounds discussed above (i.e., phentolamine and phenoxybenzamine), the agents that selectively block the postsynaptic alpha-1 receptors (doxazosin, prazosin, and terazosin) do not prevent alpha-2-receptor stimulation. Hemodynamically, the alpha-1-receptor antagonists reduce arterial pressure as a result of a fall in total peripheral resistance without an associated reflex increase in heart rate, cardiac output, or myocardial contractility. They may produce postural hypotension, often after the first dose is administered. This is said to be more common with prazosin than following the two more recently introduced agents. As a result, treatment is frequently initiated with the lowest dose at bedtime with instructions to the patient not to arise, if possible, for four to six hours. Symptomatic orthostatic hypotension is more usual one to three hours after the initial dose. With more prolonged treatment, higher doses may be required, but this may be associated with a greater potential for orthostatic hypotension. Moreover, intravascular volume expansion may occur; this will be associated with the pseudotolerance phenomenon described above. This latter problem can be offset by the addition of a diuretic; however, this may only exacerbate the former potential for postural hypotension. Other agents belonging to this class of drugs not marketed in the United States include indoramin and trimazosin.

Recently, these alpha$_1$-adrenergic receptor antagonists have been introduced for the treatment of obstructive uropathy secondary to benign prostatic hyperplasia. In these patients, particular care must be made when the alpha-1-adrenergic inhibitor is prescribed to ascertain whether the patient is already taking other antihypertensive drugs. In this case, the likelihood of postural hypotension and related symptoms is obviously increased. Furthermore, since these patients are usually older and already have nocturia secondary to the prostatic hyperplasia, the patients must be instructed to arise in gradual phases (from supine to sitting to standing) in a purposeful effort to prevent postural hypotension, falls, and fractures. At present, a new alpha receptor type 1A receptor inhibitor has been introduced (tamsalosin) which does not reduce arterial pressure but acts to relax smooth cells in the prostate thereby ameliorating symptoms without reducing blood pressure. These compounds may be of particular value for normotensive patients with benign prostatic hyperplasia.

DIRECT SMOOTH MUSCLE VASODILATORS

With the introduction of beta-adrenergic blocking therapy there was a resurgence in interest in direct-acting smooth muscle vasodilating drugs for hypertension. Moreover, these agents have been used with varying success in patients with cardiac failure. Hydralazine [Apresoline] and minoxidil [Loniten] act by decreasing arteriolar resistance. With the fall in total peripheral resistance and arterial pressure, there is a reflex stimulation of the heart so that tachycardia and palpitations (from increased myocardial contractility) frequently result unless these cardiac reflexive responses are offset by an adrenergic inhibitor (e.g., beta-blocking drug). For this reason, these agents should not be administered to hypertensive patients with myocardial infarction, angina pectoris, cardiac failure, or dissecting aortic aneurysm, because the reflexive cardiac effects of increasing heart rate, cardiac output, myocardial contractility, and the shear rate of aortic blood flow will exacerbate these underlying cardiac conditions. Other side effects include headaches and nasal stuffiness, attributable to the local vasodilation and fluid retention and edema (i.e., pseudotolerance) which occurs more frequently with minoxidil. One unique side effect of hydralazine is precipitation of a lupus erythematosus-like syndrome which occurs more frequently in patients receiving more than 400 mg/day. A common side effect from minoxidil is hirsutism, which is particularly bothersome to women. When hydralazine is administered by injection (10 to 15 mg intravenously), there is a prompt reduction in pressure. Another parenteral direct-acting smooth muscle vasodilator, diazoxide, is a non-natriuretic thiazide congener that must be injected rapidly (in single-bolus doses of 300 mg or in successive pulsed bolus divided doses) in order to prevent intravascular binding with circulating albumin in the blood. Diazoxide also should not be administered to the hypertensive patient with cardiac failure, angina pectoris, myocardial infarction, or an actively dissecting aortic aneurysm, for the reasons described above. It is, however, of value for the patient with acute hypertensive encephalopathy, intracranial hemorrhage, and severe malignant or accelerated hypertension (without cardiac failure), in whom rapid and immediate reduction in arterial pressure is mandatory.

Sodium nitroprusside, also an injectable direct-acting smooth muscle vasodilator, is very useful in hypertensive emergencies. This agent, infused by microdrip (60 μg/ml), instantly reduces arterial pressure; as the infusion rate is decreased, pressure rapidly returns to pretreatment levels. Since the agent produces venular as well as arteriolar dilation, there is less venous return to the heart and less increase in heart rate and cardiac output, and cardiac preload is diminished along with afterload. The drug therefore has particular value in treating severely hypertensive patients having myocardial infarction, cardiac failure (even with acute pulmonary edema), or dissecting aneurysm. The drug is metabolized to thiocyanate; and thiocyanate toxicity may become manifest with prolonged infusion requiring the monitoring of blood thiocyanate levels in these severely sick hypertensive patients.

ANGIOTENSIN-CONVERTING ENZYME (ACE) INHIBITORS

This class of antihypertensive agents is also effective as monotherapy for hypertensive patients of all degrees of severity, including refractory hypertension and patients with left ventricular hypertrophy, angina pectoris, and cardiac failure. These agents reduce arterial pressure by inhibiting the generation of the hemodynamically active octapeptide angiotensin II from its inactive decapeptide angiotensin I. Inhibition of ACE, therefore, inhibits both the formation of angiotensin II as well as the degradation of the active, naturally occurring, potent vasodilator bradykinin. ACE, therefore, is the same enzyme that inactivates bradykinin. Furthermore, since angiotensin II interacts with the adrenergic neurohormone norepinephrine in certain brain centers as well as at peripheral nerve endings, less angiotensin II may be available for that action. This may explain why reflexive cardiac stimulation is not generally recognized with these agents, although there does not seem to be other evidence of impaired neural reflexes. Several investigators have suggested that there also is an increased availability of prostacyclin with ACE inhibition and that the role of increased levels of circulating kinins may be important clinically in the overall antihypertensive action of these compounds. The bradykinin and angiotensin II also appear to have opposite effects in the endothelial cell. Thus, bradykinin stimulates production of that local endothelial vasodilating agent nitric oxide, and angiotensin II seems to have an opposite effect. Recent studies have demonstrated that the entire renin-angiotensin system (with the possible exception of renin itself) exists in the vascular wall and in the cardiac myocyte. These new findings provide some reasoning to explain the effectiveness of these compounds in patients with normal and low plasma renin activity and, perhaps, even in patients following nephrectomy. Hemodynamically, these agents reduce arterial pressure as a result of arteriolar dilation and a reduced total peripheral resistance; and heart rate and cardiac output do not increase reflexively. Renal blood flow usually increase in association with the reduced renal vascular resistance. Since glomerular filtration rate usually remains stable, the renal filtration fraction diminishes, suggesting that the reduced glomerular hydrostatic pressure (reported experimentally in genetic forms of hypertension by renal micropuncture studies) results from efferent as well as afferent glomerular arteriolar dilation. These effects provide an understanding for the recent reports of the value of ACE inhibitors in patients with proteinuria associated with diabetic renal disease.

ACE inhibitors are effective in patients with low and normal plasma renin activity as well as in patients with renin-dependent forms of hypertension. In this regard, they have great value in hypertensive patients with either (a) unilateral renal arterial disease with one normally functioning kidney, (b) congestive heart failure, or (c) high-renin forms of essential hypertension. They are useful as monotherapeutic agents, and their effectiveness is enhanced with the addition of a diuretic; recent reports also suggest their effectiveness when employed with calcium antagonists. And, recent evidence suggests that those agents promote arterial dilation via their endothelial action, prevent development of cardiac failure when given following myocardial infarction; and also remodel the ventricle following myocardial infarction.

There is a large number of ACE inhibitors available: captopril, enalapril, lisinopril, moexipril, quinapril, ramipril, and trandolapril. Although there may be pharmacodynamic and pharmacokinetic differences or even in their effects on the local tissue renin-angiotensin systems, they are nevertheless quite similar in their clinical effects. The ACE inhibitors have a remarkably low incidence of side effects. This is in contrast to the initial reports with captopril which suggested that leukopenia and proteinuria should be sought for during the first few months of therapy. Since then, long-term studies which included patients with less severe and less complicated forms of hypertension have indicated that these effects occur more likely in patients with impaired renal function prior to therapy or in those who were receiving immunosuppressive therapy for other diseases. Other side effects associated with ACE inhibitors include rash and cough (ascribed to the inhibited degradation of the kinins or other substances) which disappear following cessation of therapy. Angioneurotic edema following ACE inhibitors is an absolute contraindication to further ACE therapy; these agents are strictly contraindicated in pregnancy. Other problems less frequently encountered with the ACE inhibitors include sexual dysfunction and gastrointestinal side effects. As a result, an improved "quality of life" has been ascribed to these agents.

Because of its effects on other intrarenal homeostatic mechanisms (e.g., prostaglandins and kinins), treatment with ACE inhibitors may exacerbate renal functional impairment and elevate arterial pressure in patients with bilateral renal arterial disease or in patients with a solitary kidney who have unilateral renal arterial disease. Additionally, these agents should be used with extreme caution in conjunction with supplemental potassium therapy (or with potassium-retaining agents) since severe hyperkalemia may result as a consequence of reduced aldosterone.

The dry, unproductive cough seems to occur in approximately 8 to 13 percent of patients; there is no real difference among the ACE inhibitors with this effect. Not all patients with this side effect feel that it is bothersome enough to warrant discontinuation of the medication. When the drug is discontinued, it most likely will reappear when challenged again with that compound or another ACE inhibitor. If the blood pressure response to this class of agents was remarkably successful with ACE monotherapy, it would be wise to substitute the ACE inhibitor with an angiotensin II receptor antagonist (see below). The mechanism underlying cough has been explained on the basis of increased kinins resulting from inhibition of the ACE which also inhibits degradation of bradykinin. Presumably, it is the effect of kinins on pulmonary receptors that initiates the cough mechanism. Since angiotensin II antagonists act by competitive antagonism at the receptor level and not by action on the converting enzyme, justification for the use of the receptor antagonist in lieu of the ACE inhibitor is warranted. More recent studies have suggested another mechanism involving thromboxane in which thromboxane inhibitors may also modify the ACE-inhibitor induced cough. Still other studies suggest that patients within the same family who have cough association with ACE inhibitors may be on a gene-related basis. However, at this point the precise mechanisms remain unexplained.

ANGIOTENSIN II RECEPTOR ANTAGONISTS

Recent research has indicated that angiotensin II exerts its action on vascular smooth muscle, heart, kidney, adrenal cortex, brain, and other end-organs by angiotensin II receptor stimulation. Several types of angiotensin II receptors have been identified, and a specific orally active type 1 (AT-1) receptor antagonist has been synthesized which is now available (as losarten, valsarten, irbesarten) for the treatment of hypertension. Other compounds of this type and action are also under active clinical study and, presumably, will be available clinically in the very near future. Specifically, these agents exert their effects by antagonizing the angiotensin II type 1 receptors, thereby serving to attenuate the actions of angiotensin-II primarily at the vessel wall and heart. Losarten is available and effective in 50- and 100-mg doses, and most patients that respond to this agent do so in the 50-mg dosage form. As with other agents that inhibit the renin-angiotensin system, its effect is enhanced with the addition of a diuretic. A fixed combination of the two agents is also available.

In those patients who respond, the pressure reduction is mediated though a fall in total peripheral resistance with heart rate, cardiac output, and myocardial contractility not increasing reflexively in response to the pressure reduction. Early studies suggest that the agent also reduces efferent as well as afferent glomerular arteriolar resistances with associated reduction in glomerular hydrostatic pressure similar to the effects of ACE inhibition; the agent also reduces left ventricular mass. At present a number of studies are ongoing with losarten to determine its value in patients with these target organ involvements from hypertension. However, for the present, the most logical indications for the drug are in patients who developed cough with the ACE inhibitor or who, for whatever other reason, cannot take this latter class of agents.

CALCIUM ANTAGONISTS

These agents have been available for study and clinical use for at least 30 years. As a class of antihypertensive agents they are without a doubt the most heterogeneous in their chemical structure, modes of action, and clinical indications—more so than the beta-adrenergic receptor blocking agents, the actions of which are far more homogeneous. Nevertheless, the calcium antagonists have a certain commonality of action physiologically: inhibition of the availability of calcium ions in cardiac and vascular smooth muscle cells, thereby inhibiting the myocyte contractility. At least four receptors to the calcium channels have been cloned, each being responsive to calcium antagonist inhibition. This may explain some of the heterogeneity of this class of drugs in chemical structure, their pharmacological action, their physiological differences, and the potential for synergism when two calcium antagonists are used concomitantly. In addition, these agents may also differ in their intracellular actions (on release of the calcium ion from the sarcoplasmic reticulum and the mitochondria as well as binding with specific intracellular proteins (e.g., calmodulin). As arteriolar resistance is diminished, total peripheral resistance and arterial pressure falls. But even with this apparent commonality of mechanism of action, one agent (i.e., nimodipine) has little effect on total peripheral resistance and, consequently, reduction of arterial pressure; its efficacy has been shown primarily for patients with cerebral bleeding.

Nine calcium antagonists are currently available in the United States; a number of others are available elsewhere or their approval by the FDA is imminent. Verapamil, in addition to its vasodilating property, has a cardiac inhibitory action to diminish conduction and transmission. For this reason, it was used initially for the treatment of supraventricular tachyarrhythmias. In contrast, nifedipine primarily has a peripheral action to dilate arterioles; its cardiac effects are secondary to reflex stimulation of the heart as a result of the arterial pressure induction (particularly with short-acting formulation). The longer-acting formulations of this latter compound are associated with less reflex cardiac stimulation and less pedal and dependent edema. The short-acting capsular formulation of nifedipine has never been approved for the treatment of hypertension in the United States, and its use for other situations (e.g., angina pectoris) is unwise. Diltiazem (and the other agents) have actions that are intermediate, having less cardioinhibitory effects than verapamil, although there may be some reflex stimulation. All calcium antagonists reduce pressure without a consequent expansion of intravascular volume; therefore, they may be used as monotherapy for the treatment of hypertension. In part, this action is enhanced by the natriuretic effect of these agents as a result of their ability to inhibit renal tubular sodium reabsorption. As suggested above, some of these compounds (primarily nifedipine and the shorter-acting formulations of these agents) have been associated with pedal edema related to the pressure reduction. However, it must be emphasized that this alteration in fluid distribution is probably related to post-capillary reflex venoconstriction and increased hydrostatic pressure that favors trans-capillary migration of fluid into extravascular tissue. Indeed, active fluid retention on a renal basis is a highly unlikely explanation for the edema formation, and the natriuretic effect of these agents has been well documented.

As indicated, all calcium antagonists have great similarity in their antihypertensive action (except for nimodipine), which is related to a decreased total peripheral resis-tance. The reduction in vascular resistance seems to be distributed, for the most part, throughout the organ vasculatures, with the target organs of hypertension—heart, brain, and kidney—sharing in this effect. The reduced vascular resistances in these organs may also be associated with increased organ flows (depending upon the agent). All agents appear to increase coronary blood flow, but diltiazem and nitrendipine (and, perhaps, verapamil) also increase renal blood flow (probably through afferent and ef-ferent glomerular dilation) without increasing glomerular filtration rate. These agents have also been shown to maintain glomerular filtration rate and, hence, they reduce re-nal filtration fraction, hemodynamic findings that are not unlike those shown with the ACE inhibitors, although not operative through inhibition of the renin-angiotensin sys-tem. Indeed, renal micropuncture studies in various forms of experimental hyperten-sion have demonstrated efferent glomerular arteriolar dilation and reduced glomerular hydrostatic presence with diltiazem. Most calcium antagonists reduce cardiac mass (as do the ACE inhibitors), although the significance of this effect (particularly in reducing the independent risk of left ventricular hypertrophy) remains to be shown. This will be discussed in detail in Chapter 7 concerning patients with cardiac complications. The calcium antagonists have been reported to be more efficacious in volume-dependent hypertensive patients with lower plasma renin activity. Consequently, they have been recommended for older patients and black patients with hypertension. Others, includ-ing the JNC-V and JNC-VI reports, stress that these agents are also very useful in young and white patients. Because there are no metabolic side effects (e.g., hypokalemia, car-bohydrate intolerance, hyperlipidemia, hyperuricemia) associated with these com-pounds, they may be used in patients who have had these biochemical alterations with other antihypertensive agents (e.g., diuretics), and they have not been associated with sexual dysfunction. One new calcium antagonist, mibefradil, is somewhat different from those of the verapamil and diltiazem or the dihydropyridine groups in that it an-tagonizes T-channel receptor sites and does not slow heart rate. Further experience with this agent will no doubt point to clearer indications for the selection of this agent in con-trast with the other calcium antagonists. Other calcium antagonists available in the United States include: amlodipine, felodipine, isradipine, nicardipine.

A recent report has appeared detailing the results of the Syst-Eur Study in Europe. In this study a calcium antagonist of the dihydropyridine group (i.e., nitrendipine, a compound not available in the United States) was compared with placebo treatment in patients with isolated systolic hypertension in the elderly. In that study, nitrendi-pine was found to provide significant protection against stroke although upwards of 25 percent of the patients received a diuretic and many patients also received an ACE-inhibitor. Side effects related to the calcium antagonists have been constipation (pri-marily with verapamil) and flushing and headaches (with the hydropyridine com-pounds). Finally, gingival hyperplasia has been noted with most of these agents.

A brief word is in order concerning the recent controversy that has arisen from reports concerning a possibly greater likelihood of myocardial infarction in patients with hypertension treated with three short-acting formulations of nifedipine, verapamil, or diltiazem. The issue arose from a retrospective case study involving over 300 patients receiving these drugs who were compared with over 2000 patients not receiving these antihypertensive agents. In part, the study reflects the drawbacks of retrospective case studies and not the benefits of randomly assigned patients to a double-blind prospective study. In part, the results reflect the fact that the case study group of patients had a greater prevalence of complications from hypertensive and atherosclerotic vascular events prior to the initiation of antihypertensive therapy. But perhaps more important to the use of calcium antagonists was the fact that only short-acting formulations of the drugs were used; these agents, particularly the capsular formulation of nifedipine, were not even approved for use in patients with hypertension. Subsequent meta-analyses were reported confirming that the short-acting formulation of nifedipine (as opposed to the other two compounds) can produce an increased rate of myocardial infarction whether because the patients taking these medications were more predisposed to the complication or not. Thus, it seems wise to conclude at this time that short-acting formulations of calcium antagonists (and, in particular, nifedipine) are not indicated for the treatment of hypertension and that there is no reason to exclude the longer-acting formulations for the treatment of patients with hypertension.

THERAPEUTIC CONCEPTS AND CONTROVERSIES

Having covered the specific pharmacological and physiological issues dealing with the various classes of antihypertensive agents, how they interact in antagonizing clinically operative pressor mechanisms, and their unwanted effects, it is important now to consider some of the issues that exist concerning their selection in patients with hypertension and certain areas where controversy may exist. For examples, concerns have been raised by several authorities about primary prevention of hypertension, the "preference" of diuretics and beta-adrenergic receptor inhibitors for initial therapy, and the issue concerning morbidity and mortality associated with coronary heart disease. Other issues relate to the selection of antihypertensive therapy for specialized patient groups with various demographic and specific comorbid or other clinical abnormalities will be considered in subsequent chapters.

Primary Prevention of Essential Hypertension

When the first of the JNC reports was published in 1972, 23 million Americans who were believed to have essential hypertension (i.e., defined as having diastolic pressures in excess of 104 mmHg). Following publication of the results of the Hypertension Detection and Follow-Up Program, the number of potential patients with less severe essential hypertension (i.e., diastolic pressures 90 through 104 mmHg) deemed to be at risk from elevated pressures was increased to 59 million. Moreover, with publication of the Joint National Committee's third report (JNC-3), specific nonpharmacological treatment recommendations were made, including weight reduction, dietary sodium restriction, and moderation of ethanol intake. These recommendations have been revised subsequently in JNC-V and JNC-VI; but most importantly, they were rapidly accepted and implemented into the daily American lifestyle by the general public. The consequences of this overall acceptance by the public were reflected in the results of NHANES-III (National Health and Nutrition Examination Survey) that indicated the number of potential patients with essential hypertension in the United States had fallen by 16 percent to 43 million. Thus, it became dramatically apparent that the concept of the primary prevention of essential hypertension is eminently feasible and practicable. Moreover, it underscores the need to expend further efforts in emphasizing lifestyle modifications for the prevention as well as treatment of essential hypertension and its effects on coronary heart disease risk. Furthermore, we know that these measures will ensure that even if these interventions are employed in conjunction with pharmacotherapy, a significant reduction in numbers as well as doses of antihypertensive drugs that must be prescribed for a specific patient will result.

Concept of Reduced Morbidity and Mortality

Until publication of JNC-V and JNC-VI, the concept that certain antihypertensive agents significantly reduce total and cardiovascular morbidity and mortality had not been emphasized adequately. Much had been said in the earlier JNC reports about the efficacy of antihypertensive drug therapy and of its potential to reduce deaths and disability related to hypertension. However, this potential had not been stated forcefully enough and with appropriate qualifications. Thus, a specific statement was made in JNC-V that the diuretics and beta blockers "are preferred because a reduction in morbidity and mortality has been demonstrated, and that the other classes of antihypertensive agents had not yet been tested nor shown to reduce morbidity and mortality." This language led many to erroneously infer that only the diuretics and beta blockers should be recommended for initial therapy of hypertension. To the contrary, this statement was made to highlight the wealth of clinical and epidemiological data that had been generated demonstrating that only the diuretics and beta-adrenergic receptor blockers had, indeed, shown a significantly reduced incidence of fatal and nonfatal strokes, myocardial infarction, congestive heart failure, accelerated and malignant hypertension, as well as progression of hypertensive disease to stages of greater severity. Moreover, the statement is supported further by data from the European Working Party Study in which elderly patients with diastolic hypertension were treated with diuretics and methyldopa; other studies of elderly patients with diastolic hypertension supported the original meta-analyses demonstrating reduction of deaths from stroke and coronary heart disease. More recently, these findings were reinforced by other reports demonstrating that diuretics and beta blockers were also effective in reducing morbidity and mortality in elderly patients with isolated systolic hypertension in these multicenter studies. The comments concerning drug preference, while not specifically using the term "preference" is implied in JNC-VI. However, there is a reference in its recommendations for initial treatment of hypertension to the findings with the calcium antagonist nitrendipine in reducing deaths and morbidity from stroke in the recently reported Syst-Eur Study involving patients with isolated systolic hypertension in the elderly. A word of caution, however, is necessary. Nitrendipine belongs to the chemical grouping of dihydropyridine calcium antagonists; but, this entire class of drugs is so heterogeneous, it would be inappropriate to transfer the findings with nitrendipine to any of the other dihydropyridine calcium antagonists. Notwithstanding, all long-acting dihydropyridines are said in NCV-VI to have a compelling indication for isolated systolic hypertension (in older persons).

It is most important at this juncture to emphasize that each of the other classes of antihypertensive agents included in the recommendations for initial therapy in JNC-V and JNC-VI (i.e., ACE inhibitors, calcium antagonists, Angiotensin II (type 1) antagonists) alpha$_1$-adrenergic receptor and alpha-beta-adrenergic receptor blockers) have been shown to be equally effective in reducing and controlling elevated arterial pressure. However, at this time none of these other classes of antihypertensive agents have been tested in appropriately controlled multicenter studies of hypertensive patients to demonstrate the reduced morbidity and mortality from hypertension that was demonstrated with the diuretics and beta blockers. Indeed, such a study [ALLHAT (Antihypertension and Lipid Lowering Treatment for Prevention of Heart Attack Trials)] sponsored by the National Heart, Lung, and Blood Institute is presently in progress. Already, one multicenter study (the Syst-Eur from Europe) has demonstrated a reduction in stroke with the calcium antagonist nitrendipine. Another study, from China, with a less clear-cut design (the PRAISE study), using long-acting nifedipine, showed similar results in preventing stroke. It is also necessary to make clear that the JNC-V and JNC-VI reports were eminently flexible in its recommendations for the selection of initial therapy for the treatment of hypertension. (Indeed, this is the concept of this book and is emphasized in subsequent chapters.) Thus, if the physician believes that any agent from the other three or four classes of antihypertensive drugs is more suitable for a given patient, then that selection is not only appropriate and is not only recommended, but is endorsed and encouraged. Therefore, in selecting any single agent for initial treatment of hypertension, great flexibility is afforded the clinician in selection of agents for the initial treatment of hypertension.

ANNOTATED BIBLIOGRAPHY

The first two references are for JNC-V and JNC-VI, the basis for our current National guidelines for the treatment of hypertension.

Joint National Committee on the Detection, Evaluation, and Treatment of Blood Pressure: The 1992 Report of the Joint National Committee on the Detection, Evaluation, and Treatment of Blood Pressure (JNC-V). *Arch Intern Med* 1993;153: 154–183.

Joint National Committee on the Detection, Evaluation, and Treatment of High Blood Pressure. The sixth report of the Joint National Committee on prevention, detection, evaluation, and treatment of high blood pressure. *Arch Intern Med.* 1997;157:2413–2446.

Gurwitz JH, Bohn RL, Glynn RJ, Monane M, Mogun H, Avorn J: Antihypertensive drug therapy and the initiation of treatment for diabetes mellitus. *Ann Intern Med* 1992;118:273–278.

Siscovick DS, Raghunathan TE, Psaty BM, Koepsell TD, Wicklund KG, Lin X, Cobb L, Rautaharu PM, Copass MK, Wagner EH: Diuretic therapy for hypertension and the risk of primary cardiac arrest. *N Engl J Med*;1994;330:1852–1857.

The above are two excellent meta-analytic studies demonstrating the safety of low dose thiazides with respect to sudden death and diabetes mellitus.

The next eight references provide comprehensive review with lengthy bibliographies in various classes of antihypertenisve therapics.

Frohlich, ED: Diuretics in hypertension. *J Hypertens* 1987;5(Suppl 3):S43–S49.

Frohlich ED: Inhibition of adrenergic function in the treatment of hypertension. *Arch Intern Med* 1974;133:1033–1048.

Frohlich ED: Methyldopa: Mechanisms and treatment: 25 years later. *Arch Intern Med* 1980;140:954–959.

Frohlich ED: Beta-adrenergic blockade in the circulatory regulation of hyperkinetic states. *Am J Cardiol* 1971;27:195–199.

Frohlich ED: Beta-adrenergic receptor blockade in the treatment of essential hypertension. In: *The Heart in Hypertension* (Strauer BE, ed). Springer-Verlag, Berlin, 1981, 425–435.

Aristizabal D, Frohlich ED: Calcium antagonists. In: *Cardiovascular Pharmacology and Therapeutics* (Singh BN, Dzau V, Vanhoutte PM, Woosley RL, eds). Churchill Livingstone, New York, 1993, 185–202.

Frohlich ED, Angiotensin converting enzyme inhibitors: Present and future. *Hypertension* 13:125–130, 1989.

Frohlich ED, Iwata R, Sasaki O: Clinical and physiological significance of local tissue renin-angiotensin systems. *Am J Med* 1989;887:19S–23S.

Frohlich ED: Hypertension. In: *Conn's Current Therapy* (Rakel RE, ed), WB Saunders, Philadelphia, 1993, 280–296.

Frohlich ED: Hypertension: Essential. *In: Current Therapy in Cardiovascular Disease,* 4th ed. (Hurst JW, ed). Mosby–Year Book, Philadelphia, 1994, 291–299.
    The two previous references provide a concept of current antihypertensive drug therapy advocated by the author.

Frohlich ED: The United States Joint National Committee's Recommendations: Its Fifth Report (1992). In: *Textbook of Hypertension* (Swales JD, ed). Blackwell Scientific Publications, Oxford, 1994, 1203–1210.
    A review of the various national programs advocating initial therapy of hypertension.

Laragh JH, Brenner BM, ed. *Hypertension: Pathophysiology, Diagnosis, and Management.* New York, Raven Press, 1995.

Kaplan NM: *Clinical Hypertension,* 7th Edition, Baltimore, Williams & Wilkins, 1998, 444.
    The two previous references are the two current and comprehensive textbooks on hypertension.

Collins R. Peto R, MacMahon S, et al: Blood pressure, stroke and coronary heart disease. II: Short-term reductions in blood pressure: Overview of randomized drug trials in their epidemiological context. *Lancet* 1990;335:827–838.

Thijs L, Fagard R, Lijnen P, Staessen J, VanHoot R, Amery A: A meta-analysis of outcome trials in elderly hypertensives. *J Hypertens* 1992;10:1103–1109.
    The two previous references provide the current meta-analyses of the early and most recent multicenter trials of antihypertensive therapy.

SHEP Cooperative Research Group. Prevention of stroke by antihypertensive drug treatment in older persons with isolated systolic hypertension. *JAMA* 1991;265:3255–3264.

MRC Working Party. Medical Research Council trial of treatment of hypertension in older adults: principal results. *BMJ* 1992;304:405–412.

Dahlof B, Lindholm LH, Hansson L, Schersten B, Ekhom T, Wester PO: Morbidity and mortality in the Swedish Trial in Old Patients with Hypertension (STOP-Hypertension). *Lancet* 1991;338:1281–1285.
    The previous five references provide the supporting data that indicated the feasibility and rationale for the treatment of isolated systolic hypertnension in the elderly.

SECTION III

SPECIAL CIRCUMSTANCES AND DEMOGRAPHIC CONSIDERATIONS

Chapter 5

Uncomplicated Essential Hypertension

NATIONAL TREATMENT RECOMMENDATIONS

Treatment of patients with essential hypertension has been tremendously successful ever since the publication of the landmark Veterans Administrative Cooperative Study reports. With this impetus, a proscribed protocol was drafted by the Joint Coordinating Committee (JNC) of the National High Blood Pressure Education Program (NHBPEP) that was very similar to the stepped care approach developed by the VA Cooperative Studies. It was this protocol that was recommended by the first Joint National Committee (JNC) of the NHBPEP in the United States in 1972. The most recent of these reports (JNC-VI) was released in 1997. These JNC reports have been accepted broadly by primary care as well as other groups of physicians, and they are of particular value for the treatment of the patient with uncomplicated essential hypertension. Although the recommendations of these JNC reports have been quite specific, they are also highly flexible, with suggestions for other patients with essential hypertension having complications and target organ involvement, and for patients with comorbid diseases or other cardiovascular risk factors. Moreover, they are also applicable for patients with other (secondary) forms of systemic arterial hypertension.

Following publication of JNC-I the NHBPEP learned that only one-half of all people with hypertension were aware that their blood pressures were elevated. Of those people who were aware that they had hypertension, one-half of them were treated with antihypertensive therapy; and one-half of these people had their pressures under control. Thus, only 12.5 percent of our population with hypertension had their blood pressure controlled. Over the ensuing years there was much progress in the awareness, treatment and control of high blood pressure. However, with the recent publication of JNC-VI there has been an alarming concern that the numbers of those people with hypertension who were detected, treated and controlled have not improved (if not even diminished) to 68, 54, and 27 percent, respectively. The lesson from this national public and professional education program is clear: we are not doing a good job at all in our efforts to control this major cardiovascular disease and risk factor underlying coronary heart disease; and we must improve on our responsibilities. To this end, this book is dedicated.

Participating in the formulation of these JNC reports have been representatives from the JCC. These individuals are appointed by 38 professional organizations and 7 governmental organizations that are totally committed to a well-considered national approach for the identification, evaluation, management, and treatment of patients with the hypertensive diseases. Consequently, the membership of the JNC is comprised of individuals representing such professional organizations as the

American and National Medical Associations, American College of Cardiology, American Heart Association and its Council for High Blood Pressure Research, American Society of Hypertension, American College of Physicians, American College of Chest Physicians, National Kidney Foundation, the Endocrine Society, American Diabetes Association, and many other groups representing the medical, nursing, podiatric, pharmacy, and hospital management professions as well as the American Hospital Association, American Red Cross, and other groups.

In addition to disseminating these JNC reports, the NHBPEP has organized and promulgated working group reports concerned with specific problems related to hypertension. Among the more recent publications are those concerned with the heart in hypertension, stroke and hypertension, the kidney in hypertension, hypertension and diabetes, hypertension in the elderly, hypertension in the pediatric patient, nonpharmacological treatment of hypertension, the primary prevention of hypertension, adherence problems in hypertension, hypertension in the work setting, and many others. Each report has been an important resource document for all health care professional as well as for community and third-party reimbursement organizations. For specific information concerning these reports the interested reader is referred to the National High Blood Pressure Education Program, Office of Prevention, Education & Control, Department of Health and Human Services, National Institutes of Health, 31 Center Drive, MSC 2480, Building 31, Bethesda, Maryland, 20892-2480, USA.

Because of the remarkably broad acceptance of these JNC reports by primary care and other physicians in the United States, other national hypertension groups have been organized throughout the world and have disseminated their own reports to suit their own specific national needs. Such reports have been developed by national committees in Great Britain, Canada, New Zealand, and Australia, among other nations. Further, the World Health Organization (in cooperation with the International Society of Hypertension) has also developed its own document. These reports have also been published in the peer-reviewed world literature.

CURRENT TREATMENT RECOMMENDATIONS

Treatment of Stage I and II Hypertension

Patients with stage I hypertension (systolic pressures ranging from 140 through 159 mmHg or diastolic pressures from 90 through 99 mmHg), having been documented on at least three separate occasions, should have their elevated pressures brought under control. In those patients with low-grade diastolic pressure elevation (e.g., 90 through 94 mmHg), this may be approached initially with lifestyle (i.e., nonpharmacological) modifications as already described (Chapter 3). However, if the elevated diastolic pressure is not reduced within a reasonable time period (e.g., perhaps after six months), certainly less if the pressure elevation is associated with target organ involvement or a strong family history of premature death and disability, then (in my opinion), selection of antihypertensive drug treatment is clearly indicated. Indeed, this concept has been recommended in JNC-VI. By target organ involvement, I refer to clinical evidence of cardiac enlargement, cardiac failure, renal functional impairment or proteinuria, hypertensive retinopathic changes, and transient ischemic attacks or stroke (recently termed "brain attack"). In these individuals, particularly if the patient is black, older, a man, or if the hypertension is coexistent with other comorbid diseases such as carbohydrate intolerance

Table 5.1. Factors Which Favor Initiating Pharmacological Therapy in Patients with Borderline or Stage 1 Hypertension (Systolic Pressures Between 140 and 159 mmHg, Diastolic Pressures Between 90 and 99 mmHg)

1. Positive family history of cardiovascular disease with premature death
2. Failure of pressure to respond to lifestyle modifications
3. Evidence of target organ involvement
   a. Heart
      1. Left ventricular hypertrophy
      2. Cardiac failure
   b. Kidney
      1. Renal functional impairment
      2. Persistent proteinuria
   c. Brain
      1. Hypertensive retinopathy
      2. Transient ischemic attacks
      3. Stroke
4. Related co-morbid diseases or cardiovascular risk factors
   a. Carbohydrate intolerance/diabetes mellitus
   b. Hyperlipidemias
   c. Exogenous obesity
   d. Atherosclerosis
5. Significant demographic factors
   a. Male gender
   b. Black race

or diabetes mellitus, obesity, cigarette smoking, hyperlipidemia, and atherosclerosis, vigorous antihypertensive treatment should be actively employed (Table 5.1).

In those patients with Stage 2 hypertension (i.e., in whom systolic pressures are between 160 and 179 mmHg or diastolic pressures are between 100 and 109 mmHg), pharmacological therapy should be initiated at the outset together with specific and detailed advice to modify abnormal lifestyle practices (especially if other risk factors are already present). Ultimately, in these individuals, it is reasonable to withdraw antihypertensive drug therapy slowly after blood pressure has come under control for a significant period of time (one to two years), particularly when those abnormal lifestyle practices seem to have been corrected. As indicated in Chapter 3, many studies have demonstrated not only that lifestyle modification measures provide control of low-grade pressure elevations but also that in those patients with higher pressure elevations, these lifestyle changes will reduce the number of drugs (or their doses) that have been prescribed. By the same token, other studies have demonstrated that most patients with hypertension who have discontinued antihypertensive therapy must resume pharmacological therapy after its discontinuation.

CURRENT CONSIDERATIONS FOR SELECTING INITIAL THERAPY

Nonpharmacological (Lifestyle Modification) Approaches

Ever since publication of JNC-III, nonpharmacological approaches have been recommended as a basis upon which all further (pharmacological) therapy is prescribed. Studies have demonstrated that with weight control (to ideal body weight levels), sodium restriction (< 100 mEq daily), and alcohol moderation (< 1 ounce ethanol or its equiv-alents), pressure might be fully controlled in those patients with lesser degrees of systolic and diastolic pressure elevation. Subsequently, smoking cessation and a regular program of isotonic exercise have been recommended and it is reasonable to maintain these healthful practices indefinitely. A recent meta-analysis has suggested that potassium sup-plementation is effective in reducing pressure, particularly in patients with less severe hypertension or with excess sodium intake. (Further discussion of these and other non-pharmacological therapy or lifestyle modifications may be found in Chapter 3.)

Diuretic   The thiazide diuretic has been recommended for initial pharmacological monotherapy of hypertension from the very first JNC report in 1972. The rationale for this "first step" was not based solely on clinical empiricism, but also on a sound phys-iological rationale. Thus, at the time of JNC-I, the only other classes of antihyperten-sive agents that were available were the adrenergic inhibitors and the direct-acting vascular smooth muscle relaxants. Were antihypertensive treatment to be initiated with either of these two therapeutic drug classes, following an initial reduction in ar-terial pressure, there would be a return of pressure toward or to pretreatment levels—not because of drug tolerance to these agents but because intravascular volume would expand as a consequence of pressure reduction with these agents. Moreover, monotherapy with the diuretic was already known to have its intrinsic ability to re-duce arterial pressure in about 50 percent of patients with essential hypertension. With the addition of the other ("second" or "third step") classes of antihypertensive agents effective control of arterial pressure could be expected in upwards of 85 percent of treated patients; under these circumstances, lower doses of the nondiuretic agents could be employed. This therapeutic maneuver would serve to reduce the chances of developing side effects from these other agents. Thus, it was not that drug tolerance was being prevented with thiazide diuretics, but that the phenomenon of "pseudotol-erance" or the reduced effectiveness of antihypertensive therapy was the consequence of intravascular (i.e., plasma) volume expansion. Finally, and equally important, use of the diuretic with other classes of antihypertensive therapy potentiated the antihy-pertensive effectiveness of the other antihypertensive agents prescribed.

Beta-Adrenergic Receptor Inhibitors   The next class of antihypertensive agents that was recommended as an initial therapeutic option for antihypertensive monotherapy was the beta-adrenergic receptor blocking compounds (the "beta-blockers"). This class of agents was recommended as an alternative approach in JNC-III, although JNC-II had already suggested the alternate possibility. This recommendation was made because abundant experience had been amassed to indicate that beta-blockers could be prescribed for ini-tial therapy without the likelihood for intravascular volume expansion, loss of control of arterial pressure, and with predicted effectiveness in a significant population of hyper-tensive patients. Moreover, antihypertensive effectiveness of the beta-blockers was in-creased further with the addition of a diuretic agent. Therefore, even if the beta-blocker was not effective for monotherapy (e.g., in the black patient), co-treatment with a diuretic was equally effective (e.g., as when both compounds were employed in white patients).

Calcium Antagonists   While not listed in JNC-VI as preferred treatment for all patients with hypertension requiring drug therapy, recent controlled multicenter trials have indi-cated that certain calcium antagonists are of proven value in treatment of elderly patients with isolated systolic hypertension. Thus, nitrendipine (not available in the United States) was shown to reduce mortality from strokes with the Syst-Eur Study and long-acting nifedipine in the STONE Trial. The former study was well-controlled but the latter apparently has been criticized in its design. Hence, while it may be premature to suggest that all calcium antagonists are preferred for initial treatment, recent data of well-designed outcome trails are beginning to indicate their value. Many other ongoing trials employing calcium antagonists are in progress and their findings will be critically important. It was because of the results of the Syst-Eur Study that JNC-VI included the "long-acting dihydropyridine calcium antagonists nitrendipine" as a "compelling indication" for the treatment of isolated systolic hypertension (in older persons). Personally, since this group is very heterogeneous (see Chapter 4), I believe this recommendation is too all-inclusive.

Less Than Full Doses Another feature in the evolution of recommendations of initial antihypertensive therapy was made in JNC-III. This was advanced with the suggestion that therapy with either the diuretic or beta-blocker could be initiated in less than full doses. Experience over these past three (or more) decades has taught us that it was not necessary to prescribe the thiazide diuretic (e.g., hydrochlorothiazide) as 50 mg (or more) twice daily alone or with the full dose of the various beta-blocker (e.g., atenolol 100 mg daily). A significant number of patients would be expected to respond to less than full doses (e.g., 12.5 to 25 mg) of hydrochlorothiazide alone or with 25 to 50 mg of atenolol with fewer side effects.

Additional First Step Options The angiotensin-converting enzyme (ACE) inhibitors had already received considerable attention when JNC-III was published. Indeed, that report indicated that this class of agents might be suitable for initial monotherapy. Furthermore, intravascular (i.e., plasma) volume expansion was also known to be absent with these agents even though addition of a diuretic further enhanced their effectiveness.

Since JNC-V, a number of well-controlled multicenter double-blinded trials with ACE inhibitors have been shown to reduce morbidity and mortality in patients with myocardial infarction. In addition, they have been shown to prevent (or at least reduce the prevalence) of congestive heart failure following myocardial infarction. These studies have primarily been concerned with normotensive patients, however, and thus should not be extended to all patients with hypertension.

When JNC-IV was published, the two newer classes of antihypertensive agents, the ACE inhibitors and calcium antagonists, were added to the original initial options for antihypertensive therapy, the diuretics and beta-blockers. Each of these four options for initial therapy was recommended for use in less than full doses with the suggestion that these doses could be increased before adding a second pharmacological agent to the treatment program. The alpha$_1$-adrenergic receptor inhibitors and the alpha$_1$-beta receptor inhibitors were added in JNC-V and the angiotensin II (type 1) receptor blockers were added in JNC-VI.

RECENT JNC RECOMMENDATIONS

In the present set of recommendations, made in JNC-V and JNC-VI, the evolution of antihypertensive therapy has advanced further. Once again, non-drug therapies or lifestyle modifications have continued to remain the firm basis for all treatment whether they are used alone or in conjunction with drug therapy. Added to the earlier nonpharmacological modalities are smoking cessation and a regular program of dynamic exercise. (The rationale for each of these factors, along with some discussion about the other approaches presently recommended, has already been discussed in Chapter 3.)

Alpha-1 Adrenergic and Alpha-Beta Adrenergic Receptor Inhibitors

Although suggested in earlier JNC reports as possibilities for initial therapy, the $alpha_1$ adrenergic receptor and the alpha-beta adrenergic receptor inhibitors are now recommended for initial monotherapy of hypertension. These agents are effective in controlling arterial pressure with minimal intravascular volume expansion. Moreover, they were included because of approval of this class of agents by the Food and Drug Administration in the United States for the treatment of men with symptomatic benign prostatic hyperplasia. Thus, were these agents to be used by these patients with frequent nocturia, who may already be treated for hypertension with other antihypertensive agents, the addition of an $alpha_1$-adrenergic receptor blocker might predispose these patients to further blood pressure reduction or postural hypotension, as well as falls and possible bone fractures. Thus, it might be possible to prevent such potential untoward events while acknowledging effectiveness of this monotherapeutic class. A new class of $alpha_{1A}$ adrenergic inhibitors has been made available for patients with benign prostatic hyperplasia which does not reduce arterial pressure. This, obviously, will have special implications for normotensive patients or patients with hypertension in whom postural hypotension secondary to alpha receptor inhibition has been of some concern.

Other Antihypertensive Drug Classes and Drug Combinations

Since publication of JNC-V the **angiotensin II (type 1) receptor antagonists** have been approved for the initial treatment of patients with hypertension; and, currently, three are available for prescription. For this reason this class of agents has been included in JNC-VI with those agents that are appropriate for the initial treatment of hypertension. At the present time, the major indication of these agents is for those patients who had taken an ACE inhibitor and found intolerable cough. The angiotensin II receptor antagonists do not produce cough since they do not work through ACE inhibition and the increase of kinin (which may be the mechanism producing the cough). A number of studies are in progress at this time directed at certain indications including the treatment of cardiac failure, reversal of left ventricular hypertrophy, and renal involvement (related to diabetes mellitus and hypertension). At the time of this publication, there are no results available concerned with patients with hypertension.

In addition, JNC-VI cites a number of low-dose drug combinations (e.g., thiazide diuretic and potassium-sparing agent, beta-blocker and diuretic, ACE inhibitor or angiotensin II receptor antagonist and diuretic, calcium antagonist and ACE inhibitor, methyldopa or clonidine and diuretic, prazosin and diuretic, and others) as appropriate therapies for certain "compelling indications" in the initial treatment of patients with hypertension.

Concept of Reducing Morbidity and Mortality

The JNC-V committee was cognizant that the efficacy of antihypertensive therapy to reduce total and cardiovascular morbidity and mortality had not been sufficiently emphasized in prior decision-making processes for selecting initial options for monotherapy of hypertension. Furthermore, this concept is of particular relevance in these times when disease outcome events resulting from therapeutic intervention are becoming important in formulating treatment algorithms. This is very important even though much had been highlighted earlier about the efficacy of antihypertensive therapy and its potential to reduce deaths and disability related to hypertension and its complications. For this reason the following statement was included in JNC-V for initial therapy and this concept is reiterated in JNC-VI (Figure 5.1):

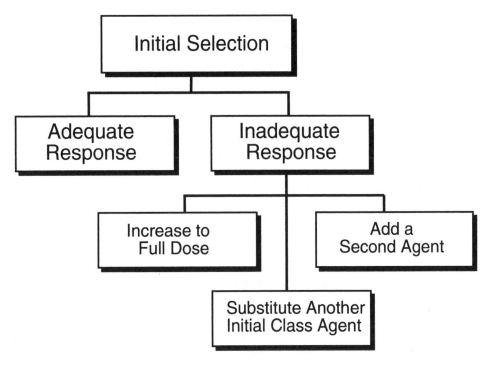

Figure 5.1. The fundamental concept for the JNC-V and JNC-VI guidelines for initial therapy of hypertension.

> "Diuretics or Beta-Blockers are preferred because a reduction in morbidity and mortality has been demonstrated. ACE inhibitors, calcium antagonists, alpha-1 receptor blockers and the alpha-beta blockers have not been tested not shown to reduce morbidity and mortality."

As indicated in Chapter 4, the rationale for stating that the diuretics and beta-blockers were preferred was to emphasize the tremendous body of epidemiological data that had accumulated over more than two decades that had demonstrated that the significant reduction in fatal and nonfatal strokes, myocardial infarction, congestive heart failure, development of accelerated and malignant hypertension, and progression in severity of hypertensive disease. Moreover, these findings have been reinforced subsequently by reports of the efficacy of these two classes of drugs in reducing morbidity and mortality in elderly patients with isolated systolic hypertension (Systolic Hypertension in the Elderly Program, from the United States; Medical Research Council Trial from Great Britain; and the STOP-Hypertension Trial, from Sweden).

This is not to say that the other five classes of agents are not as effective in reducing and controlling the elevated arterial pressure in hypertension; they certainly are. However, reductions of morbidity and mortality from hypertension had not yet been demonstrated with those five classes of agents for a variety of reasons, not the least of which are ethical and cost reasons as well as more complicated trials using positive controls. Thus, it must be emphasized that if the physician believes that employment of any of the other four classes of antihypertensive agents would be more beneficial for the patient or if other clinical and therapeutic considerations exist, selection from those other classes are clearly appropriate. This rationale may include a simpler treatment protocol, consideration of prior responses to antihypertensive therapy, the patient's overall medical status including comorbid diseases and cardiovascular risk factors, side effects of the "preferable" agents, and simplification in patient management (including the need for other drugs, laboratory tests, and missed time from work). The newest algorithm for JNC-VI is presented in Figure 5.2.

Individualization of Therapy   In providing a rationale for selecting initial monotherapy for hypertension, the JNC-V and JNC-VI reports include a detailed listing and discussion of each of the classes of antihypertensive agents, their usual dosages, mechanisms of action with pertinent comments about the actions, comparative efficacy, side effects, and contraindications (Tables 5.2 through 5.6). Indeed, the following chapters of this volume will expand in detail on these latter points, particularly with respect to the demographic characteristics of patients, hypertensive complications, and comorbid diseases.

It is well known that diuretics have certain metabolic side effects: hypokalemia, carbohydrate intolerance, some degree of reduction in renal excretory function, hyperuricemia, hypercalcemia, and, more controversially, hyperlipidemia. Each of these alterations had been identified in the earlier and more recent multicenter studies that demonstrated reduced morbidity and mortality. However, it should also be noted that in those earlier studies, the diuretics were prescribed in much higher doses than those employed in the more recent trials and that are currently recommended. Thus, the dose of hydrochlorothiazide (as an example) was recommended as 50 mg twice daily in the earlier reports; but more recently and currently the initial recommended dose is 12.5 to 25 mg daily, with the full dose as 50 mg. Using this lower dose range only minimal hypokalemia may be expected; the other metabolic alterations are less frequently experienced. Moreover, the possibility of increased total cholesterol and low-density cholesterol levels and, perhaps, lower high-density cholesterol concentration (still a subject of great controversy) is less likely to be encountered. In the final analysis, one must keep in mind that if there is any concern about development of hypokalemia, hyperlipidemia, carbohydrate intolerance or diabetes mellitus, hyperuricemia or gout or, for that matter, any other clinical concern, there are several alternatives that can be considered. First, and foremost, if there are any misgivings in employing diuretic (or other) therapy then, by all means, selection of any of the other alternative initial therapeutic classes should be made. Secondly, if these problems are not considered likely prior to initiation of therapy, measurements of these metabolic indices should be made periodically so that therapy might be then changed to an alternative agent should they occur. Similar considerations should be made with respect to the beta-adrenergic receptor blocking agents or, for that matter, any other agent initially chosen for the treatment of hypertensive disease. The information provided in Tables 5.2 through 5.6 will provide much information to assist with these decisions.

Other useful tables describe selected drug interactions (Table 5.7) and adverse effects (Table 5.8). Some of these interactions and side effects may be more familiar to the practitioner; others are less commonly encountered but are extremely important, particularly for the physician and patient encountering them. Failure (or loss) of responsiveness to antihypertensive therapy has been discussed in earlier JNC reports; Table 5.9 emphasizes some of the major considerations that should be kept in mind. Certain of the causes for loss or reduction of therapeutic responsiveness may be related to the broad professional relationship between the physician and patient: communication about the many

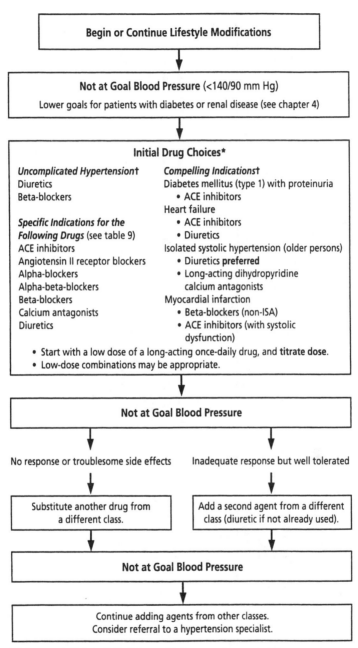

Figure 5.2. Algorithm for the treatment of patients with hypertension as presented in JNC-VI (Arch. Intern. Med. 1997; 157:2413–2446)

Table 5.2. Diuretic Agents Adapted from the Joint National Committee's 5th and 6th Reports

Diuretic	Proprietary	Dose Range (mg/day)	Frequency (times/day)	Mechanisms	Comments
Generic					
Thiazides and					
Related Agents:					
Bendroflumethiazide	Metahydrin,	2.5–5	1	Decreased extracellular (plasma) fluid volume and cardiac output initially, followed by decreased total peripheral resistance with normalization of cardiac output; long-term effects include slight decrease in extracellular fluid volume	For thiazide and loop diuretics, lower doses and dietary counseling should be used to avoid metabolic alterations
	Naturetin	12.5–50	1		More effective antihypertensives than with loop diuretics except in patients with serum creatinine ≥221 μmol/L (2.5 mg/dL)
Benzthiazide	Aquatag, Exna, Hydrex, Marazide, Proaqua	125–500	2		Hydrochlorothiazide or chlorthalidone is generally preferred; used in most clinical trials
		12.5–50			
Chlorothiazide	Diuril	1.0–2	1		
Chlorothalidone	Hygroton	12.5–50	1		
Cyclothiazide	Anhydron				
Hydrochlorothiazide	Hydro-Diuril, Esidrix	12.5–50	1		

Drug	Brand	Dose	Frequency	Comments
Microzide		2.5–5	1	
Hydroflumethiazide	Saluron	2.5–5	1	
Indapamide	Lozol	2.5–10	1	
Methyclothiazide	Enduron	0.5–1.0	1	
Metolazone	Zaroxolyn,	1.0–4	1	
	Diulo,	25.0–100	1	
Mykrox		1.0–4	1	See thiazides
Polythiazide	Renese			Higher doses of loop diuretics may be needed for patients with renal impairment or congestive heart failure
Quinethazone	Hydromox	0.5–4	2–3	
Trichlormethiazide	Naqua	25.0–100	2–3	Ethacrynic acid is only alternative for patients with allergy to thiazide and sulfur-containing diuretics
		20.0–320	2–3	
		5–100	1–2	
Loop Diuretics:				
Bumetanide	Bumex	5–10	1	
Ethacrynic acid	Edecrin	25–100	2	
Furosemide	Lasix	25–100	1	
Torsemide	Demadex			
Potassium-Sparing Agents:				
Amiloride	Midamor	Increased potassium resorption		Used mainly in combination with other diuretics to avoid or reverse hypokalemia from other diuretics
Spironolactone	Aldactone	Aldosterone antagonist		Avoid when serum creatinine ≥221 µmol/L (2.5 mg/dL)
Triamterene	Dyrenium			May cause hyperkalemia, and this may be exaggerated when combined with ACE inhibitors or potassium

Table 5.3. Beta-Adrenergic Receptor Blocking Agents Adapted from the Joint National Committee's 5th and 6th Reports

Beta Blockers Generic	Proprietary	Dose Range (mg/day)	Frequency (times/day)	Mechanisms	Comments
Atenolol*	Tenormin	25–100	1	Decreased cardiac output and increased total peripheral resistance; decreased plasma renin activity.	Selective agents also inhibit β2-receptors in higher doses (eg, all may aggravate asthma).
Betaxolol*	Kerlone	5–20	1		
Bisoprolol*	Zbeta	5–10	1		
Metoprolol*	Lopressor	50–300	1 or 2		
Metoprolol* (extended release)	Toprol	50–300	1		
Nadolol	Corgard	20–320	1		
Propranolol	Inderal	40–450	1–2		
Propranolol (long acting)	Inderal LA	60–480	1		
Timolol	Blocadren	20–60	1–2		
Esmolol	Brevibloc				only an intravenous formulation
β-Blockers with ISA:					
Acebutolol*	Sectral	200–800	1		No clear advantage for agents with ISA except in those having bradycardia who must receive a β-blocker
Carteolol	Cartrol	2.5–10	1		
Penbutolol	Levatol	10–20	1		
Pindolol	Visken	10–60	2		
α-β-Blocker:					
Carvedilol	Coreg	12.5–50	2	Same as other β-blockers, plus α$_1$-receptor blockade	Possibly more effective in blacks than other β-blockers
Labetalol	Normodyne Trandate	200–1200	2		May cause postural effects; titration should be based on supine and standing blood pressures

*Cardioselective

Table 5.4. Adrenergic Inhibitors Adapted from the Joint National Committee's 5th Report

Adrenergic Inhibitors Generic	Proprietary	Dosage Range (mg/day)	Frequency (Times/day)	Mechanisms	Comments
α₁-Receptor Blockers:					
Doxazosin	Cardura	1–16	1	Block postsynaptic α₁-receptors and cause vasodilation	All may cause postural effects; titration should be based on supine and standing blood pressure
Prazosin	Minipres	1.0–30	2 or 3		
Terazosin	Hytrin	1.0–20 (IV)	1		
α₁α₂ Receptor Blockers:					
Phentolamine	Regitine	5–10			
Phenoxybenzamine	Dibenzyline	10–40			
Centrally Acting α₂-Agonists:					
Clonidine	Catapres	0.1–1.2	2	Stimulate central α₂-receptors that inhibit efferent sympathetic activity	Clonidine patch is replaced once/wk None of these agents should be withdrawn abruptly; avoid in patients who do not adhere to treatment
Clonidine (patch)	Catapres (TTS)	0.1–0.3	1 *weekly*		
Guanabenz	Wytensin	8–32	2		
Guanfacine	Tenex	1–3	1		
Methyldopa	Aldomet	250–3000	1 or 2		
Peripheral-Acting Adrenergic Antagonists:					
Reserpine	Serpasil	0.1–0.25	1	Depletes catecholamine from neuronal storage sites	
Rauwolfia serpentina	Raudixin	50–100	1		
Alseroxylon fraction	Rauwiloid	2–4	1		
Rescinnamine	Moderil	0.25–0.50	1		
Deserpidine	Harmonyl	0.25–0.50	1		
Syrosingopine	Singoserp	1–2	1		
Guanadrel	Hylorel	10–75	2		May cause serious orthostatic and exercise-induced hypotension
Guanethidine	Ismelin	10–100	1		

Table 5.5. Angiotensin-Converting Enzyme (ACE) Inhibitors and Angiotensin II (type 1) Receptor Antagonists Adapted from the Joint National Committee's 5th and 6th Reports

Generic	Proprietary	Dosage Range (mg/day)	Frequency (times/day)	Mechanisms	Comments
ACE Inhibitors					
Benazepril	Lotensin	5.0–40	1 or 2	Block formation of angiotensin II promoting vasodilation; decreased aldosterone; also increased bradykinin and vasodilatory prostaglandins	Diuretic doses should be reduced or discontinued before starting ACE inhibitors whenever possible to prevent excessive hypotension.
Captopril	Capoten	12.5–150	2 or 3		Reduce doses in patients with serum creatinine ≥221 μmol/L (2.5 mg/dL).
Cilazapril	Inhibace	5.0–5.0	1 or 2		May cause hyperkalemia in patients with renal impairment or in those receiving potassium-sparing agents.
Enalapril	Vasotec	5.0–40	1 or 2		May precipitate acute renal failure in patients with severe bilateral renal artery stenosis or severe stenosis in artery to solitary kidney.
Fosinopril	Monopril	10.0–40	1 or 2		Contraindicated in pregnancy
Lisinopril	Zestril, Prinivil	5–40	1		Angioedema, loss of taste
Moexipril	Univasc	7.5–15	2		Leukopenia cough a common side effect
		1.0–16	1 or 2		
Perindopril	———	5.0–80	1 or 2		
Quinapril	Accupril	1.25–20	1 or 2		
Ramipril	Altace	12.5–50	1 or 2		
Spirapril	———				
Trandolapril	Mavik	1–4			
Angiotensin II (type 1) Receptor Antagonists:					
Losartan	Cozaar	25–100	1 or 2		Angioedema (very rate)
Irbesarten	Avapro	150–300	1		Hyperkalemia (as above)
Valsarten	Drovan	80–320	1		Cough not a side effect
Not Yet Approved:					
Candesarten	Biopres				
Eprosarten	Teveten				
Tasosarten					
Telmisarten					

Table 5.6. Calcium Antagonists Adapted from the Joint National Committee's 5th and 6th Reports

Calcium Antagonists Generic	Proprietary	Dosage Range (mg/day)	Frequency (times/day)	Mechanisms	Comments
Amlodipine	Norvasc	2.5-10	1	Block inward movement of calcium ion across cell membranes, reduces smooth muscle tension or produces smooth muscle relaxation	
Diltiazem	Cardizem	60-360	2-3		These agents also block slow channels in heart and may reduce sinus rate and produce heart block
Diltiazem	Cardizem-SR (sustained release)	120-360	1-2		
Diltiazem	Cardizem-CD (extended release)	120-360			
Felodipine	Plendil	2.5-20	1		Dihydropyridines are said to be more potent peripheral vasodilators than diltiazem and verapamil and may cause more dizziness, headache, flushing, peripheral edema, and tachycardia
Isradipine	DynaCirc	5-20			
Mebifradil	Posicor	50-100	2 (1 for CR)	T-channel antagonist; no further impairment of systolic function	
Nicardipine	Cardine-SR	60-90	2		Most of these agents may produce edema, flushing, headache, gingival hyperplasia
Nifedipine	Procardia-XL, Adalat CC*	30-120	1		
Nimodipine	Nimotop	For cerebral bleeding	1	Most of these agents may produce edema, flushing, headache, gingival hyperplasia	
Nisoldipine	Sular	20-60	2		Not available in U.S.
Verapamil	Calan, Isoptin, Verelon, Covera	90-480	1 or 2		
Verapamil (long-acting)	Calan SR, Isoptin SR, Covera HS	120-480	1		

*Short-acting formulation is contraindicated in hypertension

Table 5.7. Selected Drug Interactions With Antihypertensive Therapy From the Joint National Committee's 5th and 6th Reports

Diuretics

Possible situations for decreased antihypertensive effects:

- Cholestyramine and colestipol decrease absorption.
- NSAIDs (including aspirin and over-the-counter ibuprofen) may antagonize diuretic effectiveness.

Possible situations for increased antihypertensive effects:

- Combinations of thiazides (especially metolazone) with furosemide can produce profound diuresis, natriuresis, and kaliuresis in renal impairment.

Effects of diuretics on other drugs:

- Diuretics can raise serum lithium levels and increase toxicity by enhancing proximal tubular reabsorption of lithium.
- Diuretics may make it more difficult to control dyslipidemia and diabetes.

Beta-blockers

Possible situations for decreased antihypertensive effects:

- NSAIDs may decrease the effects of beta-blockers.
- Rifampin, smoking, and phenobarbital decrease serum levels of agents primarily metabolized by the liver due to enzyme induction.

Possible situations for increased antihypertensive effects:

- Cimetidine may increase serum levels of beta-blockers that are primarily metabolized by the liver due to enzyme inhibition.
- Quinidine may increase the risk of hypotension.

Effects of beta-blockers on other drugs:

- Combinations of diltiazem or verapamil with beta-blockers may have additive sinoatrial (SA) and atrioventricular (AV) node depressant effects and may also promote negative inotropic effects on the failing myocardium.
- Combination of beta-blockers and reserpine may cause marked bradycardia and syncope.
- Beta-blockers may increase serum levels of theophylline, lidocaine, and chlorpromazine due to reduced hepatic clearance.
- Nonselective beta-blockers prolong insulin-induced hypoglycemia and promote rebound hypertension due to unopposed alpha stimulation. All beta-blockers mask the adrenergically mediated symptoms of hypoglycemia and have the potential to aggravate diabetes.
- Beta-blockers may make it more difficult to control dyslipidemia.
- Phenylpropanolamine (which can be obtained over the counter in cold and diet preparations), pseudoephedrine, ephedrine, and epinephrine can cause elevations in blood pressure due to unopposed alpha-receptor-induced vasoconstriction.

ACE Inhibitors

Possible situations for decreased antihypertensive effects:

- NSAIDs (including aspirin and over-the-counter ibuprofen-like compounds) may impair blood pressure control.
- Antacids may decrease the bioavailability of ACE inhibitors.

Possible situations for increased antihypertensive effects:

- Diuretics may lead to excessive hypotensive effects (hypovolemia).

Effect of ACE inhibitors on other drugs:

- Hyperkalemia may occur with potassium supplements, potassium-sparing agents, and NSAIDs.
- ACE inhibitors may increase serum lithium levels.

Calcium Antagonists

Possible situations for decreased antihypertensive effects:

- Serum levels and antihypertensive effects of calcium antagonists may be diminished by these interactions: rifampin-verapamil; carbamazepine-diltiazem and verapamil; phenobarbital and phenytoin-verapamil.

Possible situations for increased antihypertensive effects:

- Cimetidine may increase pharmacologic effects of all calcium antagonists due to inhibition of hepatic metabolizing enzymes resulting in increased serum levels.

Effects of calcium antagonists on other drugs:

- Digoxin and carbamazepine serum levels and toxicity may be increased by verapamil and possibly by diltiazem.
- Serum levels of prazosin, quinidine, and theophylline may be increased by verapamil.
- Serum levels of cyclosporine may be increased by diltiazem, nicardipine, and verapamil. Cyclosporine dose may need to be decreased.

Alpha-blockers

Possible situations for increased antihypertensive effects:

- Concomitant antihypertensive drug therapy (especially diuretics) may increase chance of postural hypotension.

Sympatholytics

Possible situations for decreased antihypertensive effects:

- Tricyclic antidepressants may decrease the effects of centrally acting and peripheral norepinephrine depleters.
- Sympathomimetics, including over-the-counter cold and diet preparations, amphetamines, phenothiazines, and cocaine, may interfere with the antihypertensive effects of guanethidine and guanadrel.
- The severity of clonidine withdrawal reaction can be increased by beta-blockers.
- Monoamine oxidase inhibitors may prevent degradation and metabolism of norepinephrine released by tyramine-containing foods and may cause hypertension. They may also cause hypertensive reactions when combined with reserpine or guanethidine.

Effects of sympatholytics on other drugs:

- Methyldopa may increase serum lithium levels.

- This table does not include all potential drug interactions with antihypertensive drugs.

Table 5.8. Adverse Drug Effects from the Joint National Committee's 5th and 6th Reports

Drugs	Selected Side Effects	Precautious and Special Considerations
Diuretics		
Thiazides and related diuretics	Hypokalemia, hypomagnesemia, hyponatremia, hyperuricemia, hypercalcemia, hyperglycemia, hypercholesterolemia, hypertriglyceridemia, sexual dysfunction, weakness	Except for metolazone and indapamide, ineffective in renal failure (serum creatinine ≥221 µmol/L [2.5 mg/dL]); hypokalemia increases digitalis toxicity; may precipitate acute gout
Loop diuretics	Same as for thiazides except loop diuretics do not cause hypercalcemia	Effective in chronic renal failure
Potassium-sparing agents	Hyperkalemia	Danger of hyperkalemia in patients with renal failure, in patients treated with an ACE inhibitor or with NSAIDs.
Amiloride		Danger of renal calculi
Spironolactone	Gynecomastia, mastodynia, menstrual irregularities, diminished libido in males	
Triamterene		
Adrenergic inhibitors		
Beta-blockers	Bronchospasm, may aggravate peripheral arterial insufficiency, fatigue, insomnia, exacerbation of congestive heart failure, masking of symptoms of hypoglycemia. Also, hypertriglyceridemia, decreased high-density lipoprotein cholesterol (except for those drugs with ISA). Reduces exercise tolerance.	Should not be used in patients with asthma, chronic obstructive pulmonary disease (COPD), congestive heart failure with systolic dysfunction, heart block (greater than first degree), and sick sinus syndrome; use with caution in insulin-treated diabetics and patients with peripheral vascular disease; should not be discontinued abruptly in patients with ischemic heart disease.

Alpha-beta blocker Labetalol	Bronchospasm, may aggravate peripheral vascular insufficiency, orthostatic hypertension	Should not be used in patients with asthma, COPD, congestive heart failure, heart block (greater than first degree), and sick sinus syndrome; use with caution in insulin-treated diabetics and patients with peripheral vascular disease.
Alpha₁-receptor blockers	Orthostatic hypotension, syncope, weakness, palpitations, headache	Use cautiously in older patients because of orthostatic hypotension. Common: cough
ACE inhibitors		Rare: angioedema, hyperkalemia rash, ageusia (loss of taste), leukopenia Contraindicated in pregnancy. Concerns for hyperkalemia and aggravation of hypertension in patients with bilateral renal arterial disease or with unilateral disease of a solitary kidney.

Table 5.9. Causes for Lack of Responsiveness to Therapy

Nonadherence to therapy
- Cost of medication
- Instructions not clear and/or not given to the patient in writing
- Inadequate or no patient education
- Lack of involvement of the patient in the treatment plan
- Side effects of medication
- Organic brain syndrome (e.g., memory deficit)
- Inconvenient dosing

Drug-related causes
- Doses too low
- Inappropriate combinations (e.g., two centrally acting adrenergic inhibitors)
- Rapid inactivation (e.g., hydralazine)
- Drug interactions
  Nonsteroidal anti-inflammatory drugs
  Oral contraceptives
  Sympathomimetics
  Antidepressants
  Adrenal steroids
  Nasal decongestants
  Licorice-containing substances (e.g., chewing tobacco)
  Cocaine
  Cyclosporine
  Erythropoietin

Associated conditions
- Increased obesity
- Alcohol intake more than 1 ounce of ethanol a day

Secondary hypertension
- Renal insufficiency
- Renovascular hypertension
- Pheochromocytoma
- Primary aldosteronism

Volume overload
- Inadequate diuretic therapy
- Excess sodium intake
- Fluid retention from reduction of blood pressure
- Progressive renal damage

Pseudohypertension

pitfalls of the treatment and overall management program. This communication should include potential side effects, dosing instructions, and other factors that may affect drug effectiveness, including dietary sodium intake or drug interactions with over-the-counter medications. Other factors for consideration may include the cost of the therapeutic program, alternative drugs, coexistent diseases and, of course, failure to understand earlier communication. Still other therapeutic possibilities for this complex problem may relate to the medication itself (e.g., prescription of inadequate doses, inappropriate combinations of therapies, drug interactions). Always an important consideration is the need to correct "pseudotolerance" (i.e., inadequate use of diuretic therapy) or volume overload. Finally, there is need to emphasize associated disease-related problems, including more recent development of a secondary form of hypertension (e.g., atherosclerotic renal arterial disease), newer symptoms that suggest the coexistence of other secondary forms of hypertension (e.g., thyroid disease, primary aldosteronism), and problems related to associated pathological conditions, including exogenous obesity, excessive alcohol intake, and medications more recently prescribed by other physicians.

Another complex subject discussed in JNC reports has been concerned with the management of hypertensive emergencies and urgencies. Not that many years ago only a few potent antihypertensive agents were available for patients with hypertensive emergencies; the major pharmacological consideration for the use of those agents was that of reduction of arterial pressure without consideration of the specificity of drug action or associated side effect. These latter problems further complicated the overall management of the patient. Thus, effective antihypertensive agents could produce the following: paralytic ileus (from ganglionic blockers); obtunded sensorium (with reserpine); and reflexive cardiac stimulation in the patients with angina pectoris, recent myocardial infarction, or cardiac failure (with hydralazine or diazoxide). These and other concerns are emphasized in Table 5.10 which describes the variety of agents presently available, dosages, times of onset, and pertinent cautions. Consideration of this variety of critical situations may now permit the "wedding" of disease mechanisms of a specific pathophysiological hypertensive emergency with the mechanisms of drug action of the larger number of agents that are presently available (see Chapter 9).

Perhaps one of the more helpful considerations for selecting initial therapy has been the discussion that relates to the demographics, concomitant diseases and therapies, physiological and biochemical measurements, quality of life and economic considerations. Some of these had been covered in JNC-IV; but they have been presented more comprehensively in JNC-V and JNC-VI (Table 5.11). In general, the most recent JNC reports have suggested the following: Blacks (as a demographic group) may be more responsive to diuretics and calcium antagonists than to the beta-blockers or ACE inhibitors; older patients are generally responsive to all antihypertensive drug classes in contrast to what is reported in other articles in the literature and gender does not seem to dictate one form of drug responsiveness or another. It is important to remember that although the diuretics, beta-blockers, and certain calcium antagonists may be preferred, loss of efficacy can usually be overcome with the addition of a diuretic or another agent. Table 5.8 also provides a guide for the selection of specific classes of therapy for concomitant diseases, risk factors, or therapies. Review of this information may be particularly helpful in minimizing employment of excessive numbers of drugs in overall patient management. Moreover, it may obviate chances for drug interactions, side effects, and unnecessary cost of treatment. These concepts will be discussed more extensively in subsequent chapters of this book.

Subsequent Therapy Should the initial selection of therapy prove to be effective, of course, there would be no further need to add additional drugs. However, if the therapeutic response is less than optimal, there are three options to pursue: (l) the dose of the initially selected agent could be increased to its fully recommended amounts; (2) a second agent could be added to the initially selected antihypertensive agent; or (3) an alternative monotherapeutic agent may be substituted in place of the initially prescribed agent. In this regard, were the diuretic not employed initially, its addition might prove to be effective in controlling pressure as well as in reducing the dosage of the initially-prescribed agent. Moreover, it might potentiate the antihypertensive action of the initial agent, and care should be exercised without regard. Finally, the use of a second agent with a different mechanism of action than that of the initially prescribed agent is a sound concept when one considers the multifactorial nature of hypertensive disease.

Table 5.10. Management of the Hypertensive Crisis: Emergencies and Urgencies Adapted from the Joint National Committee's 5th and 6th Reports

	Dose	Onset	Cautions
Parenteral vasodilators			
Sodium nitroprusside	0.25–10 µg/kg/min as IV infusion Maximal dose for 10 minutes only	Instantaneous	Nausea, vomiting, muscle twitching; with prolonged use may cause thiocyanate intoxication, methemoglobinemia acidosis, cyanide poisoning; bags, bottles, and delivery sets must be light resistant.
Nitroglycerin	5–100 µg/min as IV infusion	2–5 min	Headache, tachycardia, vomiting, flushing, methemoglobinemia; requires special delivery system due to drug binding to PVC tubing.
Nicardipine	5–15 mg/hr (IV)	2–5	Most emergencies except cardiac failure; caution with myocardia ischemia.
Diazoxide	50–150 mg IV bolus, repeated, or 15–30 mg/min by IV infusion	1–2 minutes	Hypotension, tachycardia, aggravation of angina pectoris, nausea and vomiting, hyperglycemia with repeated injections.
Hydralazine	10–20 mg IV bolus 10–50 mg IM 10 min	10–20 min 20–30 min	Tachycardia, headache, vomiting, aggravation of angina pectoris.
Enalaprilat	0.625–1.25 mg every 6 hours IV	15–60 min	Renal failure in patients with bilateral renal artery stenosis, hypotension.
Parenteral adrenergic inhibitors			
Phentolamine	5–15 mg IV bolus	1–2 min	Tachycardia, orthostatic hypotension.
Trimethaphan camsylate	1–4 mg/min as IV infusion	1–5 min	Paresis of bowel and bladder, orthostatic hypotension, blurred vision, dry mouth.

Labetalol	20–80 mg IV bolus every 10 min; 2 mg/min IV infusion	5–10 min	Bronchoconstriction, heart block, orthostatic hypotension.
Esmolol	250–500 mg/kg/min for 1 min then 50–100 µg/kg/min (may be in repeated sequences)	1–2 min	Bronchospasm, heart block
Methyldopate	250–500 mg IV infusion every 6 hours	30–60 min	Drowsiness.
Dopamine (D_1) receptor antagonist			
Fenoldopam	0.1–0.3 µg/kg/min IV infusion	< 5 min	Tachycardia, headache, nausea, flushing; caution with glaucoma.
Oral agents			
Clonidine	0.1–0.2 mg PO, repeated every hour as required to a total dose of 0.6 mg	30–60 min	Hypotension, drowsiness, dry mouth.
Labetalol	200–400 mg PO, repeat every 2–3 hours	30 min–2 hours	Bronchoconstriction, heart block, orthostatic hypotension.

Note: It is sometimes appropriate to administer a diuretic agent with any of the above.

Table 5.11. Antihypertensive Drug Therapy: Individualization Based on Special Considerations (Modified from the Joint National Committee's 5th and 6th Reports)

Clinical Situation	Compelling Indications	Requires Special Monitoring	Relatively or Absolutely Contraindicated
Cardiovascular:			
Angina pectoris	Beta-blockers; Calcium antagonists		Direct vasodilators
Bradycardia/Heart block, Sick sinus syndrome			Beta-blockers; Labetalol; Verapamil; Diltiazem
Cardiac failure	Diuretics; ACE inhibitors		Beta-blockers; Calcium antagonists; Labetalol
Myocardial infarction	Beta-Blockers (non-ISA), ACE Inhibitors		
Hypertrophic cardiomyopathy with severe diastolic dysfunction	Beta-blockers; Diltiazem; Verapamil		Diuretics; ACE inhibitors; Alpha$_1$-blockers; Hydralazine; Minoxidil
Isolated systolic hypertension (elderly)	Diuretics, certain calcium antagonists		
Hyperdynamic circulation	Beta-blockers		Direct vasodilators
Peripheral vascular occlusive disease			Beta-blockers
Postmyocardial infarction	Non-ISA Beta-blockers; ACE inhibitors		Direct vasodilators
Renal:			
Bilateral renal arterial disease or severe stenosis in artery to solitary kidney			ACE inhibitors
Renal insufficiency			
Advanced (serum creatinine ≥221 µmol/L [2.5 mg/dL])	Loop diuretics	ACE inhibitors	Potassium-sparing agents Potassium supplements

Other:

Condition			
Asthma/COPD			Beta-blockers; Labetalol
Cyclosporine-induced hypertension	Calcium antagonists, Labetalol		Verapamil*; Diltiazem*; Nicardipine*
Depression			Alpha$_2$-agonists Reserpine
Diabetes mellitus Type I (insulin dependent)	With proteinuria-ACE inhibitors, certain calcium antagonists may have a favorable response.		Beta-blockers Beta-blockers; Diuretics
Dyslipidemia	alpha-blockers (may be of value) beta-blockers, some calcium antagonists	Diuretics; Beta-blockers	
Liver disease		Labetalol	Methyldopa
Benign prostatic hyperplasia	alpha-blockers		
Vascular headache	Beta-blockers		
Pregnancy Preeclampsia Chronic hypertension	Methyldopa; Hydralazine Methyldopa		Diuretics; ACE inhibitors ACE inhibitors

*May increase serum levels of cyclosporine.

Other Considerations Among other areas highlighted in JNC-V were the findings concerned with the treatment of isolated systolic hypertension, particularly in elderly patients. This therapeutic advance was restated in JNC-VI and has been discussed above with respect to preference of diuretic and beta-blocker therapy for initial treatment and, earlier, with the inclusion of systolic pressure elevation in considering the staging (or severity) of hypertensive disease. Also highlighted was a discussion of "step-down therapy," a therapeutic maneuver that is directed toward reduction in doses or numbers of agents employed in an overall antihypertensive treatment program. Inherent in this concept is the continued adherence to lifestyle modifications. Indeed, this approach is particularly sound for those patients who have effectively followed a program of proscribed lifestyle modifications which had served not only to control arterial pressure but to diminish risk factors predisposing that patient to premature cardiovascular disease and death. After reducing the dosages of different agents, the drugs to be withdrawn from the therapeutic program are those deemed less necessary to provide optimal control of pressure. Clearly, agents that are useful in also treating other diseases should be retained for the coincident treatment of hypertension.

Finally, as in the earlier reports, the more recent JNC reports included discussion concerning the frequency and number of follow-up visits, guidelines for patient educational programs, and strategies to improve adherence to therapy and for control of high blood pressure.

In conclusion, the series of JNC reports have provided yet another practical example of the evolution of antihypertensive therapy. The recommendations have reflected the increasing sophistication in our knowledge about the pathophysiology of the hypertensive diseases and their complications as well as the increasing variety and greater specificity of the agents that continue to become available for selection of antihypertensive therapy. These reports have demonstrated the value of sound, but nonrigid and modifiable guidelines for the treatment of hypertension. In that regard, it is less important to be concerned of a formed therapeutic algorithm; rather, the overriding concern should be how to select our first step in the overall pharmacological management program should be in a specific patient.

SUGGESTED READINGS

References 1 through 7 are the major national guidelines (world-wide) for the treatment of hypertension.

1. Joint National Committee on Detection, Evaluation, and Treatment of High Blood Pressure. The 1992 Report of the Joint National Committee on Detection, Evaluation, and Treatment of High Blood Pressure (JNC-V). *Arch Intern Med,* 1993;153:154–583.

2. Joint National Committee on Detection, Evaluation, and Treatment of High Blood Pressure. The 1996 Report of the Joint National Committee on Detection, Evaluation, and Treatment of High Blood Pressure (JNC-VI). *Intern Med,* 1997; 157:2413–2446.

3. Sever P, Beevers G, Bulpitt C, Lever A, Ramsay L, Reid J, Swales J. British Hypertension Society Second Working Party Report. Management guidelines in essential hypertension. *BMJ* 1993;306:983–987.

4. Ogilvie RI, Burgess E, Cusson J, Feldman R, Leiter L, Myers M. Recommendations for the pharmacological treatment of essential hypertension: Report of the Canadian Hypertension Society Conference Committee on treatment. *Can Med Assoc J* 1993; 149:575–584.

5. Hypertension Guidelines Committee. Hypertension, diagnosis, treatment and maintenance. Guidelines endorsed by the High Blood Pressure Research Council of Australia. Royal Australian College of General Practitioners, Adelaide, Australia, 1991.

6. National Advisory Committee on Core Health and Disability Support Services. *The Management of Raised Blood Pressure in New Zealand.* National Advisory Committee on Core Health and Disability Support Services, Wellington, New Zealand, 1992.

7. Guidelines Subcommittee. 1993 Guidelines for the management of mild hypertension: Memorandum for a WHO/ISH meeting. *J Hypertens* 1993;11:905–918.
References 1–6 are specific national (and international) efforts to provide rationale in prescribing practices for the treatment of hypertension.
References 8 and 9 were the first landmark publications by the Veterans Administration Cooperative Study on Antihypertensive Agents that established the efficacy of antihypertensive therapy and a simple protocol for treatment.

8. Veterans Administration Cooperative Study Group on Antihypertension Agents. Effects of treatment on morbidity in hypertension. I. Results in patients with diastolic blood pressure averaging 115 through 129 mmHg. *JAMA* 1967;202: 1028–1034.

9. Veterans Administration Cooperative Study Group on Antihypertensive Agents. Effects of treatment on morbidity in hypertension. II. Results in patients with diastolic blood pressure averaging 90 through 114 mmHg. *JAMA* 1970;213: 1143–1152.
References 10–12 demonstrated the value of nondrug measures for controlling blood pressure.

10. Trials of Hypertension Prevention Collaborative Research Group. The effects of nonpharmacologic interventions of blood pressure of persons with high normal levels: results of the Trials of Hypertension Prevention, Phase I. *JAMA.* 1992;267: 1213–1220.

11. Treatment of Mild Hypertension Research Group. The Treatment of Mild Hypertension Study: a randomized, placebo-controlled trial of a nutritional-hygienic regimen along with various drug monotherapies. *Arch Intern Med.* 1991;151: 1413–1423.

12. Wassertheil-Smoller S, Blaufox MD, Oberman AS, Langford HG, Davis BR, Wylie-Rosett J. The Trial of Antihypertensive Interventions and Management (TAIM) study; adequate weight loss, alone and combined with drug therapy in the treatment of mild hypertension. *Arch Intern Med.* 1992;152: 131–136.
References 13–16 demonstrated the safety and efficacy of antihypertensive drug therapy for reducing morbidity and mortality of isolated systolic hypertension in the elderly.

13. SHEP Cooperative Research Group. Prevention of stroke by antihypertensive drug treatment in older persons with isolated systolic hypertension. *JAMA.* 1991;265:3255–3264.

14. MRC Working Party. Medical Research Council trial of treatment of hypertension in older adults: principal results. *Br Med J.* 1992;304:405–412.
15. Dahlöf B, Lindholm LH, Hansson L, Scherstén B, Ekbom T, Wester PO. Morbidity and mortality in the Swedish Trial in Old Patients With Hypertension (STOP-Hypertension). *Lancet.* 1991;338:1281–1285.
16. Staessen JA, Fagard R, Thijs L, et al, for the Systolic Hypertension-Europe (Syst-Eur) Trial Investigators. Morbidity and mortality in the placebo-controlled European Trial on Isolated Systolic Hypertension in the Elderly. Lancet 1997;360:757–764.

Chapter 6

Hyperdynamic Circulatory States in Hypertension

For many years, the physician has been concerned about patients whose blood pressure measurements could be defined as being consistent with hypertensive disease while at other times the blood pressure levels are consistent with what would be considered normal. Clearly, physicians who have managed the health care of these patients have been confused. This confusion has only been exceeded by that of their patients who are otherwise healthy but are, at times, said to have overall cardiovascular health that has been considered to be "at risk." This risk was established by epidemiologists and actuaries of "third parties" (i.e., health care insurance carriers) who for very pragmatic and practical reasons have found that the patients are at increased risk for premature cardiovascular morbidity and mortality. The judgment is usually made on routine physical examinations, at times of selection into military service, for employment purposes, or even for participation in formal athletic activities.

The fact of the matter is that measurement of blood pressure should be done accurately. Thus, if the blood pressure is taken as prescribed by published standards and is found to be truly elevated by an average of measurements obtained on at least three distinctly separate occasions, the diagnosis of hypertension is satisfied. The patient is then said to have systemic arterial hypertension and is at increased risk. Hence, the diagnosis is clear and the patient should be treated. However, there are many circumstances in which the diagnosis is not necessarily that clear-cut and the decision to treat the patient may be controversial. This chapter discusses some of these circumstances (Table 6.1). Because of the great variability of arterial pressure, controversy has frequently surrounded the establishment of the diagnosis of hypertension. This variability of arterial pressure is still greater the higher the level of the pressure. This great variability or fluctuation (often moment to moment) of pressure has been related to the participation of adrenergic mechanisms and the associated hemodynamic indices (e.g., arterial pressure, heart rate, cardiac output). In any event, patients are said to have established systemic arterial hypertension if either the systolic or diastolic blood pressure equals or exceeds 140 and 90 mmHg, respectively, on at least three separate occasions. Thus, the higher the averaged pressure (systolic or diastolic), the greater will be the severity staging (Table 6.2).

LABILE HYPERTENSION

For many years, physicians termed patients who were asymptomatic and otherwise "healthy" and, yet, at times had intermittently elevated diastolic pressures as having

Table 6.1. Some of the Diagnoses Used Historically for "Early" Hypertension and Hyperdynamic Circulatory States

1. Early essential hypertension
   a. "High normal" blood pressure
   b. Juvenile hypertension
   c. Prehypertension
   d. Borderline hypertension
   e. Labile hypertension
2. Borderline isolated systolic hypertension
3. Borderline isolated diastolic hypertension
4. Office ("white coat") hypertension
5. Hyperdynamic circulatory states
   a. Soldier's heart syndrome
   b. DaCosta's syndrome
   c. Irritable heart syndrome
   d. Neurocirculatory asthenia
   e. Cardiac anxiety
   f. Anxiety neurosis
   g. Hyperkinetic heart syndrome
   h. Hyperdynamic beta-adrenergic circulatory state
   j. Idiopathic mitral valve prolapse syndrome

Table 6.2. Classification of Adult Hypertension Based Upon Systolic and Diastolic Pressure Levels.[a]

Category	Systolic (mm Hg)		Diastolic (mm Hg)
Optimal	<120	and	<80
Normal	<130	and	<85
High normal	130–139	or	85–89
Hypertension			
Stage 1	140–159	or	90–99
Stage 2	160–179	or	100–109
Stage 3	≥180	or	≥110

[a]Whatever pressure level is greater (systolic or diastolic) that level confers the severity stage.

"labile hypertension." Those very patients, who at times had diastolic pressures less than 90 mmHg and at least on two other occasions had diastolic pressures equal to or greater than 90 mmHg, were studied by means of careful hemodynamic assessment in the 1960s, and their physiological characteristics were found to be different than an otherwise normal population of patients. This term "labile hypertension," however, was discontinued because, as already stated, all arterial pressure measurements are labile. In fact, the higher the level of arterial pressure, the more labile and fluctuant are the measurements and the greater will be the variance of the pressure around that level. For this reason, the term "labile hypertension" was discontinued and the term "borderline hypertension" was thereupon established for this group.

BORDERLINE HYPERTENSION

Clinically and hemodynamically, the term "borderline hypertension" was created to characterize that group of otherwise asymptomatic and normal individuals whose diastolic pressures were less than 90 mmHg, but at other times (on at least two occasions) diastolic pressure was 90 mmHg or greater. However, at that time the Framingham Heart Study also began to classify their cohort of patients according to the height of both systolic and diastolic pressures. According to that study, patients whose systolic and diastolic pressures were less than 140 and 90 mmHg, respectively, were said to be normotensive. However, if the systolic and diastolic pressures were 160 or more and 90 or more mmHg, respectively, they were said to have definite hypertension. But if the systolic and diastolic pressures fell between 140 through 159 or 90 through 94 mmHg, respectively, they were said to have either borderline systolic or borderline diastolic hypertension, respectively. It is unfortunate that this term of "borderline hypertension" has been defined differently and concurrently by these two schools of researchers, the physiologists and the epidemiologists. However, the readers of their reports can soon differentiate the differences in definition according to the context in which the term is used.

Thus, when studied hemodynamically, patients with borderline hypertension, particularly when they are younger, have a faster heart rate, an elevated cardiac output, and an increased left ventricular ejection rate and other evidence of myocardial contractility. These physiological investigators soon learned that associated with the foregoing systemic hemodynamic characteristics of a hyperdynamic circulation were increased levels of circulating norepinephrine, plasma renin activity, and urinary excretion of cyclic adenosine monophosphate—all humoral factors that are consistent with a hyperdynamic circulation that is associated with an increased adrenergic output to the cardiovascular, renal, and endocrine systems. Not only is the increased cardiac output associated with an increased chronotropic and inotropic evidence of myocardial function, but there is an augmented venous return to the heart which is the result of peripheral venoconstriction that redistributes circulating blood volume to the central circulation. This is demonstrable by a significant increase in the cardiopulmonary volume in the absence of an expanded intravascular (i.e., plasma) volume. The total peripheral resistance in these patients was found to be "normal." However, if truly normal individuals were to have an elevated cardiac output to the levels measured in these "borderline hypertensive" patients, their total peripheral resistance would actually be reduced. Hence, we suggested that the total peripheral resistance in these individuals with borderline hypertension is actually inappropriately normal. In addition to these studies, some of these patients with borderline hypertension were followed for a few decades by their physician-investigators and studied periodically by hemodynamic studies. Those patients who developed hypertension (and these were many) were then found to have a sustained elevation of diastolic pressure associated with an absolute increase in total peripheral resistance and a normal cardiac output. Thus, as the hypertensive state progresses in severity over the years, the reduction in cardiac output is proportional to the degree of contraction in the circulating intravascular (i.e., plasma) volume and an increased total peripheral resistance. Hence, there is less intravascular volume to be redistributed centrally from the peripheral circulation; and the cardiopulmonary volume, the venous return to the heart, and the cardiac output declines as vascular resistance increases. This increase in total peripheral resistance and in the component organ vascular resistances in general is proportional to the increase in arterial pressure and reduction in cardiac output and contraction of plasma volume.

From a very practical point of view, the elevated arterial pressure in patients with borderline hypertension (i.e., with intermittently elevated systolic and systolic pressures) is higher than that of an otherwise normal population and does confer an increased risk for premature cardiovascular morbidity and mortality according to life insurance actuarial data gathered over many decades. Moreover, this risk is also definitely increased in patients with borderline hypertension as defined by the Framingham Heart Study. Hence, borderline hypertension has been considered by insurance companies and other groups dependent upon these data to determine whether a greater risk exists than in otherwise normal individuals. Admittedly, it is difficult at any one time to predict which individuals with borderline hypertension: (1) will eventually develop established essential hypertension; (2) may continue to have blood pressure characteristics of borderline hypertension, or (3) may even subsequently have normotensive pressures thereafter. However, to my way of thinking, such patients—particularly if there is a strong family history of hypertension and premature morbidity and mortality from cardiovascular complications of hypertension—should be monitored very carefully with the following actions: periodic measurement of pressure; assessment of cardiac structure and function as well as of renal function; specific advice on nonpharmacological measures and lifestyle modifications; and, if pressure continues to rise, even corrective antihypertensive drug therapy. Then, even if the pressure is stage 1 on "High Normal" and other risk factors exist, therapeutic intervention is necessary.

OFFICE ("WHITE COAT") HYPERTENSION

Over the years, clinicians have frequently experienced the clinical phenomenon of patients who display much higher blood pressures when taken in their office. However, when the patient takes his own blood pressure at home with a sphygmomanometer permitting self-measurement of blood pressure, the pressures are less than 140 and 90mmHg systolic and diastolic, respectively. This phenomenon has been reinforced in more recent years with experiences using automatic and ambulatory blood pressure measurement by a variety of these portable electronic devices. Some authorities have reported that these individuals have "normal" home and ambulatory pressures and, hence, are not hypertensive. However, in my opinion (and that of other authorities), to date there are still insufficient normative data (for all age groups, both genders, and all racial groups) to permit a clear definition of just what are normal home or ambulatory blood pressures. Moreover, these "normotensive" people by ambulatory or other recorders have not been followed prospectively to determine whether they encounter a normal frequency of morbid events or mortality. Clearly, thousands of normal people have been studied and reported; but, to my way of thinking, these data do not counteract the decades of actuarial data amassed by insurance companies from hundreds of thousands (or more) of people. Thus, all long-term at-risk data have been based upon casual office blood pressure measurements obtained in the physician's office and not from self-measurement or ambulatory data not acquired in the physician's office setting. Moreover, data from the Tecumseh Blood Pressure Study (and others) have demonstrated that patients with borderline or "white coat" hypertension are at significantly greater risk of developing sustained blood pressure elevation, target organ damage from hypertensive vascular disease, and they are also at significantly greater risk for the subsequent development of coronary heart disease.

HYPERDYNAMIC BETA-ADRENERGIC CIRCULATORY STATE (AND OTHER HYPERDYNAMIC CIRCULATORY STATES)

From the very earliest descriptions as well as in Avicenna's writings, we have come to learn about the anxious patient with a rapid and bounding pulse, palpitations, widely dilated pupils, flushed and hot skin, and cardiac awareness. Moreover, over the past 100 or more years, patients have been described in the medical literature with various clinical syndromes whose clinical characteristics are remarkably similar.

The descriptions are usually that of young men who were examined by physicians at the time they were conscripted into the military service associated with wars. Thus, Da-Costa's or Soldier's Heart Syndrome was described during and after the Civil War in the United States; Soldier's Heart syndrome and neurocirculatory asthenia were described during World War I; cardiac anxiety and anxiety neurosis were described during World War II; and the hyperkinetic heart syndrome were described during the Vietnam War.

In 1966, we described patients who presented with complaints that included disturbing cardiac awareness (severe palpitations, rapid heart action), cutaneous flushing, pounding headaches, feelings of warmth with diaphoresis, and extreme variability of arterial pressure. Heart rate was disturbingly fast when the patient assumed an upright position; this finding was associated with pressure of a fist clenched deep into the abdomen (the Goetz reflex). A systolic ejection-type murmur was frequently heard on cardiac examination. On physiological and hemodynamic evaluation, the patients demonstrated evidence of a hyperdynamic circulation (with an elevated or normal arterial pressure) that was associated with an increased heart rate, cardiac output, and left ventricular ejection rate (Figure 6.1.); and there was an inappropriate increase in heart rate and reflex cardiac stimulation upon assuming the upright posture with head-up tilt. These physiological findings were associated with an increased responsiveness of heart rate to graded increasing doses of an intravenous infusion of the beta-adrenergic receptor agonist isoproterenol (Figure 6.2). Moreover, their symptoms and hyperdynamic circulatory physiological findings were controlled with specific pharmacological treatment, either intravenous or prolonged oral administration of the beta-adrenergic receptor antagonists propranolol (or similar agents) (Figure 6.3). None of these patients had evidence to support the diagnosis of pheochromocytoma, hyperthyroidism, or other clinically identifiable hyperdynamic circulatory states. Plasma catecholamine levels are not increased to levels of patients with pheochromocytoma. These patients, no doubt, are but a fraction of the overall population of patients whose arterial pressure exhibit great fluctuation ranging from normotensive to hypertension that may be unrelated to cardiovascular symptoms (including those patients with labile or borderline hypertension). However, it was of further interest that when we studied patients with borderline hypertension with evidence of an idiopathic mitral valve prolapse syndrome hemodynamically and during a similar isoproterenol syndrome (exhibited by a systolic click and evidence of prolapse echocardiographically), they also demonstrated an inappropriate increase in heart rate and systolic pressure (as compared with age- and gender-matched control subjects) and they had increased

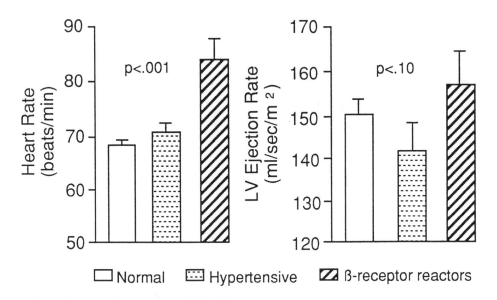

Figure 6.1 Resting supine heart rate and left ventricular ejection rate in normotensive (☐), established essential hypertensive (▦), and hyperdynamic beta-adrenergic circulatory state β-receptor reactor (▨) patients. (With permission of Frohlich ED, et al, *Arch Intern Med* 1969;123:1–7.)

circulating levels of norepinephrine. Furthermore, their symptoms, abnormal physiological findings, and mitral prolapse were all corrected with a beta-adrenergic receptor blocking drug. These findings were subsequently corroborated by others.

TREATMENT

As indicated, in general, the most advisable course of therapy in patients with borderline hypertension, office ("white coat") hypertension, or even asymptomatic hyperdynamic circulation is careful follow-up (with blood pressure measurement and monitoring for target organ structural and functional changes) and management of other cardiovascular risk factors. The latter management obviously includes intervention of all lifestyle modification modalities to minimize cardiovascular risk that could predisposes these patients to increased morbidity and mortality.

In those patients with borderline hypertension with more clear-cut evidence of target organ involvement (renal functional impairment or proteinuria, left ventricular hypertrophy or cardiac failure, history of transient ischemia attacks or strokes), institution of antihypertensive drug treatment is worthy of consideration in my opinion. I believe that this decision is valid even if arterial pressure remains "borderline" or high normal. This is particularly valid, I believe, in patients with a strong family history of hypertension with premature cardiovascular morbidity and mortality. Moreover, it's all the more pertinent if the patient is older, male, black, and has additional cardiovascular risk factors (including obesity, a history of cigarette smoking, carbohydrate

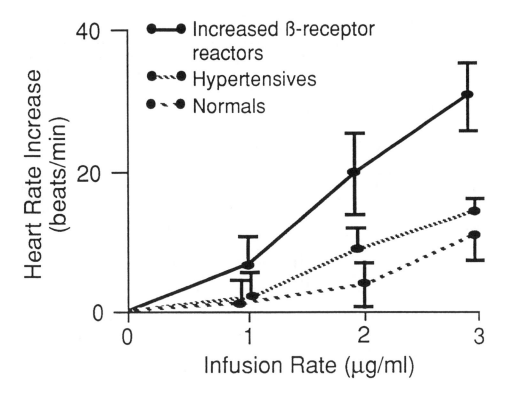

Figure 6.2 Response of heart rate to sequentially increasing intravenous infusion doses of isoproterenol in normal (●•-•●), established essential hypertensive (●•••●), and increased β-receptor reactor patients (●—●) with hyperdynamic beta-adrenergic circulatory state. (With permission of Frohlich ED, et al, *Arch Intern Med* 1969; 123:1–7).

intolerance or diabetes mellitus, hypercholesterolemia, and perhaps, hyperuricemia and hyperinsulinemia). This is supported by the recent JNC-VI recommendations if target organ involvement (e.g., left ventricular hypertrophy, proteinuria, elevated serum creatinine concentration) exists.

In those patients with severe enough cardiovascular symptoms associated with a hyperdynamic circulatory state, a beta-adrenergic blocking agent has been quite beneficial. Symptoms are alleviated and arterial pressure is controlled. If a beta blocker is contraindicated for reasons such as asthma, obstructive lung disease, depression, hypertriglyceridemia or decreased high-density hypoproteinia, or greater than a first-degree heart block, then it might be worthwhile to try a course of therapy with a centrally active adrenergic blocking agent (e.g, methyldopa or clonidine-patch), reserpine (but not in patients with depression), or, possibly even guanethidine or guanedril in lower doses.

Thus, in the final analysis, one must remember that the risk of blood pressure elevation is a continuum and that selection to initiate antihypertensive drug therapy is arbitrary and based upon long-standing and compelling actuarial data. In my opinion, the level of arterial pressure requiring treatment decreases and urgency for pharmacotherapy

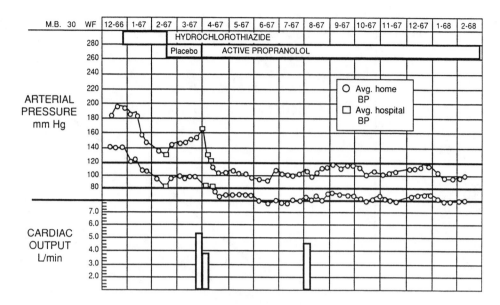

Figure 6.3 Response of a patient with hyperdynamic beta-adrenergic circulatory state to the beta-adrenergic receptor blocking agent propranolol. (With permission of Frohlich ED, et al, *Arch Intern Med* 1969;123:1–7.)

increases with the coexistence of additional cardiovascular risk factors, target organ involvement, comorbid diseases, and the patient's personal medical and family history.

ANNOTATED BIBILOGRAPHY

1. Frohlich ED, Kozul VJ, Tarazi RC, Dustan HP: Physiological comparison of labile and essential hypertension. *Circ Res* 1970;27:55–69.
2. Adamopoulos PN, Chrysanthakopoulis SG, Frohlich ED: Systolic hypertension: Nonhomogeneous diseases. *Am J Cardiol* 1975;36:697–701.
3. Frohlich ED: High cardiac output hypertensions. *Angiology* 1976;27:475–485.
4. Messerli FH, de Carvalho JGR, Christie B, Frohlich ED: Systemic and regional hemodynamics in low, normal, and high cardiac output in borderline hypertension. *Circulation* 1978;58:441–448.
   References 1–4 provide physiological data delineating the evidence that differentiates patients with labile or borderline hypertension from normal individuals.
5. Julius S, Mejia A, Jones K, Krause L, Schork N, van de Ven C, Johnson E, Petrin J, Sekkarie MA, Kjeldsen SE, Schmouder R, Gupta R, Ferraro J, Nazzaro P, Weissfeld J: White coat versus sustained borderline hypertension in Tecumseh, Michigan. *Hypertension* 1990;16:617–623.
6. Pickering TG, James GD, Boddie C, Harshfield GA, Blank S, Laragh JH: How common is white coat hypertension? *JAMA* 1988;259:225–228.
   Pro and con arguments concerning the "white coat hypertension" controversy.

References 5 and 6 present both sides of the controversy dealing with white coat hypertension. My personal feelings are expressed in the text.

7. Frohlich ED, Dustan HP, Page IH: Hyperdynamic beta-adrenergic circulatory state. *Arch Intern Med* 1966;117:614–619.

8. Frohlich ED, Tarazi RC, Dustan HP: Hyperdynamic beta-adrenergic circulatory state: Increased beta receptor responsiveness. *Arch Intern Med* 1969;123:1–7. References 7 and 8 are two initial clinical and physiological descriptions of the hyperdynamic beta-adrenergic circulatory state and are followed by two references (9 and 10) providing additional discussions on this fascinating subject.

9. Wooley CF: Where are the diseases of yesteryear? DiCosta's syndrome, soldiers' heart, the effort syndrome, neurocirculatory asthenia, and the mitral valve prolapse syndrome. *Circulation* 1976;53:749–751.

10. de Carvalho JGR, Messerli FH, Frohlich ED: Mitral valve prolapse and borderline hypertension. *Hypertension* 1979;1:518–522. Two discussions were "forms fruste" of the hyperdynamic beta-adrenergic circulating state.

Chapter 7

The Hypertensive Patient with Cardiac Complications

GENERAL

A number of cardiac derangements complicate the natural history and progressive course of systemic hypertensive vascular disease. In addition, several independent comorbid diseases, each with its respective natural history, can further complicate the overall clinical problem of hypertensive cardiac and vascular disease. One cardiac complication of essential hypertension, perhaps its most common, is that of left ventricular hypertrophy (LVH) with its attendant coronary vascular hemodynamic alterations exacerbated by increased myocardial oxygen demand, increased absolute and minimal coronary vascular resistance, reduced coronary blood flow and flow reserve, and increased blood viscosity. These adverse changes participate importantly in the complex multifactorial pathophysiology of LVH (Figure 7.1) and significantly influence the increased independent risk of LVH that accounts for its premature cardiovascular morbidity and mortality. Indeed, LVH very definitely predisposes the affected patient to microvascular angina pectoris, myocardial ischemia, fibrosis, infarction, cardiac dysrhythmias, cardiac failure, and sudden cardiac death. It is exceedingly important for the cardiovascular and primary care physician to recognize the devastating potential of those factors and comorbid diseases that are associated with LVH and hypertensive heart disease. Thus, clear recognition and understanding of the pathophysiology of LVH will permit a clearer establishment of overall diagnosis as well as an improved long-term management and more enlightened treatment of the patient. This discussion is designed to facilitate that understanding.

One important example of the coexistence of comorbid diseases relates to the frequent association of essential hypertension and LVH with occlusive (epicardial) coronary arterial atherosclerosis. Thus, hypertensive vascular disease compromises normal cardiac function through several important complications: initiation and progression of LVH; involvement of the coronary arterioles as a result of the same mechanisms that involve all of the systemic arterioles in hypertension; acute and chronic ischemic hypertensive heart disease with microvascular angina pectoris; acute and chronic left ventricular failure; ventricular dysrhythmias; and sudden cardiac death (as described above). Each of the foregoing complications exacerbate the likelihood of complications and death from occlusive atherosclerotic epicardial coronary arterial disease.

119

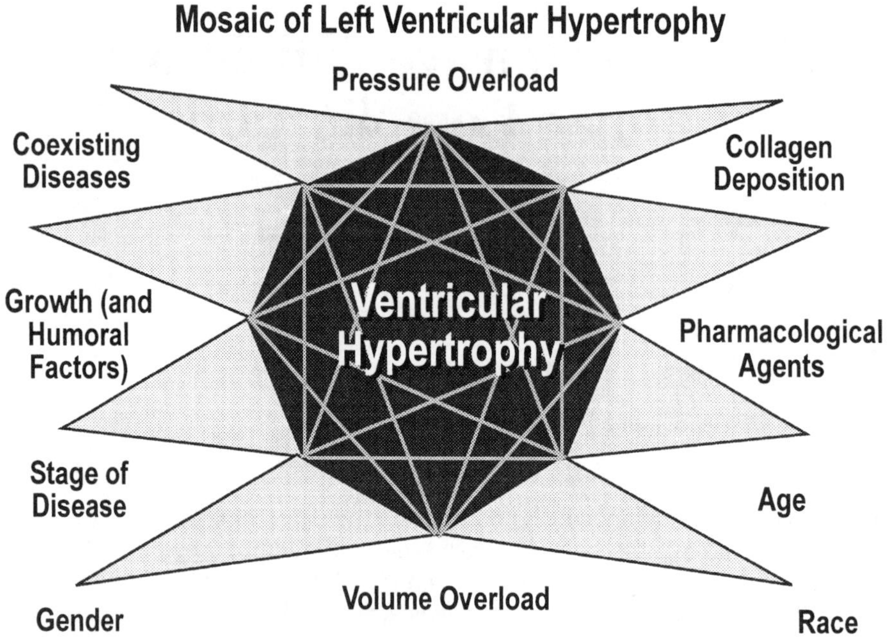

Mosaic of Left Ventricular Hypertrophy

Figure 7.1. A mosaic of LVH factors involved in the multifactorial relationships underlying the development and reversal of LVH. (with permission of the *Journal of Hypertension.*)

COMORBID DISEASES

Atherosclerosis is an independent comorbid disease process that results in occlusion of the larger epicardial coronary arteries and ischemic disease of the heart. This frequently also results in angina pectoris, myocardial ischemia, fibrosis, infarction, left ventricular failure, cardiac dysrhythmias, and sudden cardiac death. Therefore, each of the two diseases, hypertension and atherosclerosis, follows its own natural history and each accelerates, exacerbates, and is a major underlying risk factor of the other (Figure 7.2).

Diabetes mellitus frequently is associated with essential hypertension and may have its own specific cardiac and vascular complications. Diabetes also accelerates and aggravates the development and elaboration of cardiovascular disease (and is another independent and major risk factor underlying coronary heart disease). It is also associated with other cardiac and vascular complications, including those of hypertension. Diabetes impairs tissue perfusion of the major target organs (including the heart) as well as other organs by enhancing the atherosclerotic progression of disease of the medium-sized and larger coronary and other arteries and of the microcirculation of the kidneys and other organs. It, therefore, exacerbates the impaired tissue perfusion of kidney, heart, brain, eyes, and skeletal muscle which is already impaired by the arteriolar constriction and reduced blood flow and blood flow reserve of these organs from hypertensive vascular disease. In addition, diabetes accounts for a further degree of enlargement of the left ventricle at any given level of arterial pressure. Whether this is the result of more se-

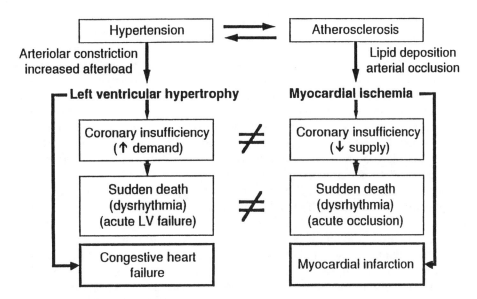

Figure 7.2. Natural histories of disease. A general concept detailing the national history of two cardiac diseases, hypertension and myocardial infarction. (With permission of *Hurst's The Heart*, 9th Ed., 1998).

vere myocardial hypertrophy or the result of augmented myocardial fibrosis or other infiltrative disease (e.g., protein deposition) remains a subject of intense study at the present time.

Still another disease that commonly coexists with hypertension is *exogenous obesity,* yet another independent risk factor underlying atherosclerosis and coronary heart disease. Obesity exacerbates hypertensive heart disease by superimposing a significant volume overload (or increased preload) upon the left ventricle through intravascular volume expansion that is in direct proportion to the increased body mass. Thus, the heart in patients with obesity and hypertension suffers from volume as well as pressure overload which, in turn, promotes a dimorphic structural adaptation, one of eccentric as well as concentric LVH.

Tobacco addiction and *hyperlipidemia* are also additional independent risk factors underlying coronary heart disease, and they also confound the complexity of hypertensive heart disease. Some of these comorbid diseases and complications will be discussed in further detail below. Moreover, other comorbid cardiac diseases may include hypertrophic cardiomyopathy, idiopathic mitral valve prolapse syndrome, myocardial fibrosis of the elderly, and impaired coronary arterial endothelial disease. And, clearly, the aging process, per se, is another complicating factor.

LEFT VENTRICULAR HYPERTROPHY

As already stated, LVH is the major cardiac complication that is directly associated with systemic arterial hypertension, ascribing a risk that is independent of the elevated arterial pressure (whether systolic or diastolic).

Hemodynamic Correlates in LVH Development

As discussed earlier, the left ventricle progressively increases its mass and wall thickness in direct proportion to the unrelenting and progressive afterload imposed upon it by the added chamber stress. Thus, while the structural changes of concentric LVH take place in response to the left ventricular afterload, they provide an efficient adaptive means for overcoming the physical forces necessary to maintain stable contractile function. This is a positive aspect of LVH in that it slows eventual left ventricular failure (unless the disease is intervened by effective antihypertensive therapy). On the other hand, this adaptive feature of LVH is offset by its intrinsic independent risk of premature cardiovascular morbidity and mortality.

Meerson suggested several decades ago that the initial response of the heart to pressure overload is that of the Frank–Starling ventricular hyperfunction. This functional response is then followed by a period of stable hyperfunction that is associated with the structural adaptation of LVH. Our hemodynamic research work has confirmed the sequence postulated by Meerson in patients with essential hypertension; we further confirmed these findings in the spontaneously hypertensive rat (SHR), which is probably the best experimental model of naturally occurring essential hypertension. Moreover, the SHR studies extended the clinical findings by providing the microcirculatory, biochemical, and histologic changes that could not otherwise be assessed clinically. Eventually, if the hypertensive patient is not adequately treated and the ventricilar afterload is not ameliorated, left ventricular failure eventually ensues. Thus, in the early years of the Framingham Heart Study, hypertension was shown to be the prime cause of left ventricular failure. And, most importantly, a more recent report from that study (in 1996) indicated that hypertension still remains as the major cause of cardiac failure in this country.

Recent Knowledge of LVH Development

In recent years, however, we have learned that the functional and structural changes described above do not necessarily occur in the sequential order initially described in Meerson's experimental pressure overload studies and later described in patients by our investigative team. Thus, recent molecular and cellular biological research has clearly shown that *simultaneous* with the increased functional performance of pressure overload hypertrophy (i.e., the stage of Frank–Starling hyperfunction), there is a concurrent biological response by the cardiac myocytes. Therefore, as the cardiac myocyte is stretched by its very earliest pressure overload, the cell is stimulated to increase its protein synthesis process and cellular hypertrophy results. Thus, the cardiac response of pressure overload is not simply functional followed by structural adaptations; both responses occur simultaneously. It is of particular interest to understand how these cellular biological responses were demonstrated. Yazaki and his associates cultured isolated cardiac myocytes from newborn rats. They then removed the cells from culture and stretched them in such a fashion that this physical stimulus provoked an early gene (i.e., the cellular proto-oncogene *c-myc*) induction which, in turn, initiated nuclear (DNA) myocytic directed protein synthesis. Therefore, the sequence that had been postulated earlier by Meerson can now be modified. Instead of the initial hyperfunctional response being followed by one of structural adaptation, the initial myocytic stretch (induced by pressure overload) evokes simultaneous hyperfunctional as well as structural adaptive responses.

Clinical Correlates of LVH Progression

In our earlier clinical investigative work, we demonstrated that one of the very early changes related to early development of LVH is that of impaired left ventricular filling during diastole. We showed that these changes can be identified clinically and electrocardiographically by the presence of an atrial diastolic gallop rhythm (i.e., fourth heart sound or bruit de galop) (Table 2.4). This long-recognized heart sound is a clinical finding that is highly concordant with electrocardiographic indices of left atrial abnormality, higher arterial pressure, and an increased prevalence of cardiac dysrhythmias. Indeed, when we first reported our initial echocardiographic study that describes the structural and functional correlates in patients with essential hypertension, those patients with only left atrial abnormality [by electrocardiogram (ECG)] had a greater left ventricular mass and thicker septal and posterior wall thickness as well as a larger left atrium. In addition, left ventricular contractility was already impaired at this stage. Furthermore, those patients with obvious LVH (by ECG) had a significantly larger left ventricle (by mass as well as wall thickness) than those patients with only left atrial abnormality; all of these patients with ECG-LVH had an enlarged left atrium by echocardiography. Hemodynamically, then, as one progresses from the normal subject to the essential hypertensive patient with atrial enlargement and then to obvious LVH, arterial pressure and total peripheral resistance increase *pari passu* and these hemodynamic changes are associated with the structurally adaptive changes of LVH.

More recent clinical investigations have shown that as LVH increases further in size, coronary hemodynamics also become progressively impaired. Thus, as the total peripheral resistance increases, it is shared uniformly in all of the component organ circulations of the systemic circulation, including the coronary arterioles. This increased coronary vascular resistance is soon associated with a reduction in the coronary blood flow and coronary blood flow reserve. Scheler and colleagues have demonstrated this hemodynamic sequence in patients with LVH without ST-segment changes, and then when LVH was associated with ST-segment deviation by measuring coronary blood flow before and after administration of the coronary vasodilatory dipyridamole (Figure 7.3). These changes may occur in patients with only hypertensive coronary arteriolar disease in the absence of atherosclerotic occlusive epicardial coronary arterial disease. Clearly, however, the ischemic disease of the myocardium is exacerbated when occlusive epicardial coronary atherosclerosis is superimposed upon hypertensive heart disease, especially when LVH is clearly present.

Nonhemodynamic Factors Underlying LVH

Over the years we have come to learn that while the hemodynamic factors of arterial pressure elevation and associated pressure and volume overload are the prime factors that trigger the development and maintenance of LVH, nonhemodynamic factors also participate importantly (Figure 7.1). Many clinical and experimental studies have provided compelling data to support this thesis. For example, while hemodynamic functions are more directly related to the structural changes of LVH in the black patient with hypertension, this does not appear to be as clear-cut in white patients. A similar body of data seems to be accumulating which suggests that development of LVH may be more severe in men than in women (most likely, through other mechanisms). Whether these factors are related to volume, hormonal, humoral, or other pressor, physiological, or growth mechanisms remains a subject of intense investigation and interest.

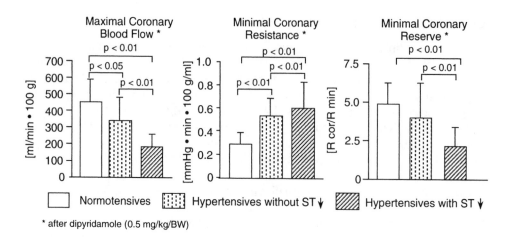

Figure 7.3. Comparison of coronary blood flow, coronary resistance, and coronary reserve in patients with hypertension and left ventricular hypertrophy (Scheler, S, et al: *Am J Cardiol* 1994;73:480).

The foregoing concept is supported by a large body of experimental data. Thus, there is a lack of correlation between the increases in arterial pressure and left ventricular mass in the laboratory model of essential hypertension, the SHR, although such a close relationship exists with the Goldblatt (two-kidney, one-clip renal) hypertensive rat. Moreover, this same functional/structural dissociation has also been shown to occur in male and female SHRs treated from conception with beta-adrenergic blocking drugs. Additionally, development of myocardial hypertrophy and increased protein synthesis has been shown when norepinephrine, isoproterenol, or angiotensin II is added to tissue culture of myocytes. Further support for this concept is offered by demonstrating induction of proto-oncogenes by these agents with subsequent expression of cellular protein synthesis.

Coexisting Pathophysiological Changes

It is well known that development of pathological LVH is associated with collagen deposition and myocardial fibrosis. Not only is this fibrosis of the ventricular wall associated with development and progression of LVH, it may also exist with occlusive coronary arterial ischemic heart disease as well as with the aging process. These changes provide support to the recent reports detailing the frequency of diastolic dysfunction in patients with hypertension. And more often than not, this occurs in patients with hypertension with LVH, coexisting occlusive epicardial atherosclerotic coronary arterial disease, or who are elderly. Each of these states is associated with impaired coronary flow reserve.

Endothelial Dysfunction

One common factor that relates to hypertensive coronary arteriolar disease, ischemic heart disease secondary to atherosclerosis, and ischemic heart disease secondary to the aging process (as well as secondary to tobacco smoking) is impaired vascular endothelial generation of nitric oxide. Nitric oxide is a naturally occurring and locally produced vasodilator synthesized from L-arginine that regulates myocardial (and other organ) blood flow. Impairment in nitric oxide synthesis by the endothelium results in increased vascular resistance and reduced local blood flow. The diminished blood flow leads to the sequelae of ischemia, fibrosis, and tissue necrosis. At present, there is much ongoing and exciting research (both experimental and clinical) focusing on the consequences and therapeutic implications of inhibited nitric oxide synthesis in disease. Since nitric oxide interacts with the local kinin-bradykinin, renin-angiotensin, and fibrinolytic systems, this new aspect of coronary hemodynamic regulation has extremely important clinical implications. This concept is all the more important since experimental studies have shown that the angiotensin converting enzyme (ACE) inhibitors as well as the angiotensin II (type 1) receptor antagonists have reversed the effects of nitric oxide synthase inhibition and increased organ (e.g., heart, kidney, and forearm) blood flows and flow reserves. In this regard, we have shown experimentally that an inhibitor of endothelial nitric oxide synthase (N^G-nitro-L-arginine methyl ester or L-NAME) mimics the local ischemic effects of hypertensive arteriolar disease and the aging process in both kidney and heart. The consequence of this L-NAME inhibition of nitric oxide synthesis is ischemia, fibrosis, intravascular thrombosis, and necrosis. Moreover, each of these pathological alterations has also been shown to be prevented or reversed by an ACE inhibitor given either with or following L-NAME administration, respectively.

Ventricular Dysfunction and Structural Changes

Myocardial (as well as renal) ischemia and fibrosis is manifested by impaired organ function. Early in the development of LVH the effects on myocardial ischemia are less evident, but systolic function is impaired first. In fact, this is why impaired systolic contractile function was first documented in the patients that we studied. These patients generally have no evidence of symptomatic ischemic myocardial disease, although systolic contractile function and resting cardiac output and renal blood flow are reduced. At this time the patients' ages range from the third to the fifth decade. However, more recently, diastolic dysfunction has been described in older patients with hypertension who obviously have coexistent ischemic heart disease secondary to the hypertension and atherosclerotic coronary arterial disease as well as aging. The pathophysiological alterations, whether by the ongoing process or by hypertensive or atherosclerotic disease, are associated with increased collagen deposition in the ventricle. This, no doubt, adds to the stiffness and reduced distensibility of the ventricular chamber, which restricts ventricular filling and contractility. Since studies in our laboratory and others have shown reduction in collagen content of the ventricle by ACE inhibitors, further credence for employment of these agents is suggested. Thus, these coexisting comorbid events have more immediate, long-standing as well as potentially preventive therapeutic implications.

From the foregoing discussion, it is clear that other common coexisting diseases and disease processes exacerbate the ischemic process whether produced by (a) reduction of coronary blood flow by vessel occlusion, (b) active arteriolar constriction, (c) impaired local endothelial regulation of myocardial flow, or (d) associated deposition of connective tissue in the ventricular wall.

Cardiac Failure

When the adaptive myocardial responses of LVH and local blood flow regulation no longer can sustain the systemic demands for cardiac output and organ blood flows, left ventricular failure supervenes. Indeed, as already indicated, hypertensive heart disease was the most common cause of cardiac failure 35 years ago in the United States, and it remains so today. When one considers that 25 years ago over 85 percent of patients with hypertension were not effectively treated and that after a generation of medical education this has been reduced to only about 60 percent, the lessons have not been conveyed clearly enough. We know that congestive heart failure can be significantly reduced with antihypertensive therapy. This was shown in the first controlled multicenter Veterans Administration Cooperative studies when only reserpine, hydralazine, and hydrochlorothiazide were available. With subsequent introduction of the beta blockers, ACE inhibitors, and calcium antagonists, reduction in the continuous increase in hospitalizations from cardiac failure is eminently possible; but this has not been observed. In the final analysis, the best way of treating LVH and cardiac failure resulting from hypertension is prevention, and early treatment of hypertension is essential; thereby, the development of LVH can be obviated in the first place. The lesson is clear: We must initiate antihypertensive therapy early enough and with effective blood pressure reduction, and control is an absolute necessity.

REVERSAL OF HYPERTROPHY

All agents that reduce arterial pressure, if used for a sufficient period of time, will reduce left ventricular mass and wall thickness and, hence, will reverse LVH. However, certain agents may reverse LVH more rapidly (even within 3 to 12 weeks) experimentally in laboratory animals and in hypertensive patients as well. This rapidity in LVH mass reduction strongly suggests that certain antihypertensive agents possess specific nonhemodynamic qualities described earlier (in the development of LVH) that may also participate in LVH reversal or its "regression."

Pharmacological LVH Reversal

The first antihypertensive agent that demonstrated true LVH reversal was methyldopa. However, these experimental studies also indicated that the LVH "regression" was not solely the result of hemodynamic "unloading" of the left ventricle. First, reversal of LVH occurred very rapidly within three weeks, and it was also associated with a reduction in the mass of the right ventricle that was neither hypertrophied nor subjected to pressure or volume overload. Moreover, both the left and right ventricular masses were reduced in the normotensive control rats; yet, surprisingly, the aortic mass was not reduced by methyldopa in either rat group. When another centrally acting adrenolytic compound (i.e., clonidine) was administered to the SHR (of the same age and gender), similar hemodynamic effects were achieved but the left ventricular mass was not reduced. Then, when the clonidine dose was tripled, producing an agonistic effect on the peripheral $alpha_1$-adrenergic receptor sites, the total peripheral resistance increased and, surprisingly, the cardiac mass decreased. These studies again demonstrated participation of non-hemodynamic factors in LVH regression.

Using the same experimental protocol that we employed with methyldopa, similar (but not identical) effects were demonstrated following administration of ACE inhibitors. Furthermore, not every ACE inhibitor produced the same structural effects as others within that drug class. Thus, while left ventricular mass was reduced in all SHR with LVH, some of these agents also reduced left ventricular mass in the normotensive rats; and none affected right ventricular mass. The effects on aortic mass was also variable in the SHR.

Our findings with calcium antagonists were similarly perplexing. Thus, while every calcium antagonist reduced the left ventricular mass of the hypertensive rats, they did not produce this effect in the normotensive rats without LVH. Furthermore, while LVH was reversed in the SHR, the right ventricular mass actually increased. This, however, was not due to developed right ventricular hypertrophy, but it resulted from increased deposition of collagen in that chamber. Moreover, this occurred as left ventricular collagen actually decreased. Furthermore, when an ACE inhibitor was given along with the calcium antagonist, the right ventricular collagen deposition was prevented, although the ACE inhibitor did not diminish the left ventricular mass and collagen content further.

The precise mechanism accounting for the rapid reduction in left ventricular mass is not yet at hand. While a common mechanism of this disparate group of pharmacological agents could be shared by less available intracellular calcium ions available for protein synthesis, it may also be related to different other mechanisms. Thus, LVH reversal may be the consequence of less generated (locally or systemically) angiotensin II and its mitogenic effects. Favoring this concept are the findings of LVH reversal associated with administration of angiotensin II (type 1) receptor antagonists. Also possible is the participation of locally generated kinins resulting from ACE inhibition; this argument may be supported by the synergistic action on both arterial pressure and LVH mass reversal by the ACE inhibitors when used together with the angiotensin II receptor antagonist (referred to earlier).

Questions may be legitimately raised as to whether pharmacologically induced LVH reversal may be associated with impaired left ventricular pumping ability as left ventricular muscle mass diminishes. This thesis may be supported teleologically by the concept that LVH is developed initially to prevent development of cardiac failure. However, with reversal of that structural adaptation, cardiac failure might be precipitated were antihypertensive therapy to be suddenly withdrawn. Actually, we tested that possibility experimentally in the SHR with LVH reversal, when arterial pressure was abruptly increased. Those left ventricular pumping ability studies revealed a Frank–Starling curve that was consistent with a failing left ventricle when methyldopa reversed LVH; however, a normal Frank–Starling curve was obtained following treatment with any of several ACE inhibitors or several calcium antagonists.

One may also question whether reversal of LVH might be associated with improved coronary hemodynamics. In our earlier studies, we measured coronary blood flow and flow reserve following LVH reversal after three weeks' treatment with the ACE inhibitors and calcium antagonists. Myocardial flow did not improve after only three weeks treatment, nor was it improved when an ACE inhibitor (i.e., enalapril) was administered for as long as 12 weeks. However, when an angiotensin II receptor antagonist (e.g., losartan) was given alone or with the same ACE inhibitor and was administered for 12 weeks, coronary blood flow and flow reserve and minimal coronary vascular resistance improved in association with the reduction in left ventricular mass.

Actually, the pressure reduction, left ventricular mass regression, and coronary hemodynamics all synergistically improved with the combination treatment. Moreover, this occurred when one-half of the dose of both agents (that had been employed alone) was administered for the 12-week treatment period.

Most of these findings obtained in the laboratory with naturally developing genetic hypertension in the SHR have been confirmed in patients with essential hypertension. Thus, reduction of left ventricular mass and wall thicknesses have been demonstrated echocardiographically within 4 to 12 weeks in patients with essential hypertension treated with centrally acting adrenergic inhibitors, beta-adrenergic receptor blocking agents, ACE inhibitors, calcium antagonists, and angiotensin II (type 1) receptor antagonists. Moreover, we also demonstrated clinically an increased right ventricular wall thickness echocardiographically within the same time period with each of seven different calcium antagonists. Moreover, studies in other laboratories have also shown improved coronary blood flow and flow reserve with long-standing ACE inhibition therapy in patients with LVH. Therefore, in summary, there appears to be a definite dissociation expressed by various antihypertensive agents with respect to their structural and hemodynamic effects in the experimental setting; early findings support this concept clinically. These differences (between various classes of agents as well as between agents within the same drug class) suggest variability among drugs in reversing LVH either through their ability to penetrate the myocyte or by their specific effects on specific myocytic biological functions.

Implications of LVH Reversal

At this time, we still do not know whether pharmacologically induced reduction of left ventricular mass (or even reversal of LVH) is associated with reduction of the increased cardiovascular risk that is conferred on the affected patient with LVH. A few recent preliminary reports have suggested this may be so; however, this assertion must be confirmed and fully established by controlled prospectively designed clinical trials. Therefore, we must clarify with absolute certainty whether the reduction in left ventricular mass (and in wall thicknesses) that is measured echocardiographically or with other technology represents true reversal of the process of cellular hypertrophy or reduction in collagen or other constitutive components of the ventricular wall. Furthermore, we must know clearly whether the reduced cardiovascular risk that may very well occur with the decreased left ventricular mass actually resulted from LVH reversal or whether that reduced risk could also be attributed to control of arterial pressure, the antiarrhythmic effects of the drugs employed, or even the direct hemodynamic coronary vascular effects that were produced by the prescribed agent, per se. I have no doubt that in the nearer rather than more distant future, these concerns will be answered by well-controlled multicenter clinical studies.

SPECIFIC THERAPEUTIC RECOMMENDATIONS

Hypertension and LVH Assessment

Clearly, the approach to the patient with essential hypertension and LVH depends upon the diagnostic means for establishing the existence of LVH. Echocardiographic technology is far better able to detect LVH than the ECG; but this methodology is not as precise as magnetic resonance imaging or other new and more costly technologies. On the other hand, the ECG is more precise than the standard posteroanterior chest roentgenogram and has the advantage of wide availability and lesser cost. In any event, as already stated, the best way to manage LVH in any asymptomatic patient with essential hypertension (no matter what technique is employed to establish its presence) is effective and careful control of arterial pressure with antihypertensive drug therapy. In my opinion, this means that the goal of arterial pressure reduction should be below 140 mmHg systolic and 90 mmHg diastolic.

At this time, the major indication for performing echocardiography is in those patients with stages I or II hypertension when the existence of LVH may be in question. If that be the case, a less costly (but less detailed) limited echocardiogram may be employed. If LVH is definitely shown by the ECG, there is little need to obtain the more costly study unless there is concern as to whether the echocardiogram will provide further information concerning left ventricular structure or function. These concerns relate to issues about contractile function, early evidence of cardiac failure, coexistent valvular heart disease, chest pain, and so on. Furthermore, there seems to be little need for the clinician to repeat an echocardiogram more frequently after one year or more.

Drug Therapy

As already stated, all antihypertensive agents may be expected to be associated with LVH reversal; this includes the diuretics and even the direct-acting smooth muscle vasodilators. The earlier JNC reports considered primarily those concepts concerning antihypertensive drug efficacy and the safety. Clinical outcome issues related to the potential of antihypertensive agents to reduce deaths and disability, but primarily to complications of hypertensive disease, were not addressed. These latter aspects of antihypertensive therapeutic clinical guidelines were approached first in JNC-V, which indicated the preference for diuretics and beta blockers and was continued in JNC-VI. As discussed earlier in greater detail, these classes of antihypertensive agents had demonstrated reduced morbidity and mortality in controlled multicenter clinical trials. This finding was contrasted with the other drug classes that had neither been tested nor shown to reduce morbidity and mortality in such trials. I believe that the discussion that ensued concerning the word "preference" wrongly inferred the concept that only the diuretics and beta blockers were recommended for initial therapy of hypertension. Use of the concept of drug "preference" (for diuretics or beta blockers) merely emphasized the compelling clinical and epidemiological data that demonstrated their ability to reduce fatal and nonfatal strokes, myocardial infarction, congestive heart failure, accelerated and malignant hypertension, dissecting aortic aneurysms, and progression of hypertensive disease to stages of greater severity.

SYSTOLIC HYPERTENSION IN THE ELDERLY

The foregoing clinical guidelines statement was supported further by data obtained from elderly patients with isolated systolic hypertension (Systolic Hypertension in the Elderly Program, MRC trial in Great Britain, and STOP-Hypertension Trial in Sweden). These patients were also treated with diuretics and beta blockers, but the doses of diuretics were much less than the doses employed in the earlier drug trials. Each of these studies demonstrated reduction in fatal and nonfatal strokes and nonfatal morbidity from coronary heart disease. However, at this point, it is most important to emphasize that each of the other four classes of antihypertensive agents are also recommended as being equally effective in reducing and controlling elevated arterial pressure. None of these other classes (or the most recent class of antihypertensive agents, the angiotensin II, type 1, receptor antagonists) have been tested thus far in controlled, multicenter trials to demonstrate reduced cardiovascular morbidity and mortality with prolonged treatment. Such a study [e.g., ALLHAT (Antihypertension and Lipid Lowering Treatment for Prevention of Heart Attack Trials)] is currently in progress and is sponsored by the National Heart Lung and Blood Institute in the United States. Therefore, if a physician believes that any one agent is more suitable for any given patient, then it is not only appropriate, but also recommended and encouraged. The major therapeutic objective at this time is well-controlled systolic and diastolic pressure.

Hence, if a diuretic or a beta-adrenergic receptor blocking agent does not control arterial pressure adequately; and, if chest pain or discomfort complicate clinical management of the patient, other antihypertensive agents may very well be indicated (*vide infra*).

CONTROVERSY CONCERNING REDUCED MORBIDITY AND MORTALITY FROM CORONARY HEART DISEASE

With respect to coronary heart disease (CHD) outcomes, recent controversy and concern has been raised by some that the diuretics might neither reverse LVH nor reduce the risk of myocardial infarction because of their potential to produce hyperlipidemia (and, thereby, to promote atherosclerosis). The TOMHS (Treatment of Mild Hypertension Study) confirmed earlier reports demonstrating that diuretics will reduce ECG indices of LVH. With respect to other clinical outcomes, much discussion had been focused in recent years on the interpretation of statistical meta-analyses of the first 14 controlled, independent, randomized multicenter trials (Figure 7.4). This analysis concluded that, although the predicted prevention of deaths from stroke (by 35 to 40 percent) had been demonstrated (actually 43 percent), the predicted prevention of deaths from CHD (20 to 25 percent) had not (i.e., 14 percent) been realized. Deaths from stroke are always demonstrated first because of the extremely positive association with elevated arterial pressure. Deaths from coronary heart disease are even more multifactorial and, once a placebo-controlled study is discontinued because deaths from stroke had been demonstrated, the biostatistical problems related to coronary heart disease are confronted. Thus, many editorial comments and other clinical reports thereupon concluded that prevention of stroke had been demonstrated by those antihypertensive drug trials, but that they *failed to prevent myocardial infarction.* However, this was neither the conclusion by the meta-analysis nor the conclusion by the actual studies.

CHD DEATHS

Actually, the above meta-analysis did not state that there was no prevention from myocardial infarction, but that the predicted decrease in deaths from *coronary heart disease* had not been achieved. Actually, a highly significant ($p < 0.001$) reduction in deaths from CHD occurred. In this respect, the term employed by the epidemiologists,

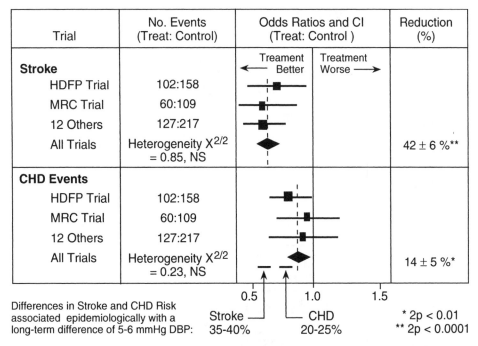

Figure 7.4. Meta-analysis concerning outcome effects of blood pressure reduction on stroke and CHD events. From the initial 14 multicenter antihypertension trials (Collins C, et al: *Lancet* 1990;335:827–838).

coronary heart disease (CHD), was not defined as being synonymous with myocardial infarction. Deaths from CHD included not only those deaths resulting from myocardial infarction, but also those resulting from lethal cardiac arrhythmias, congestive heart failure, severe angina pectoris without autopsy-proved myocardial infarction, or otherwise unexplained sudden cardiac deaths. Hence, any potential elevation in serum lipids produced by diuretics or beta blockers does not satisfy the speculation for the lack of achieving the predicted reduction in CHD deaths on the basis of exacerbated atherogenesis. First, myocardial infarction was not the sole determinant of death from CHD. Second, hyperlipidemia is not a major adverse effect with the presently recommended initial diuretic doses (i.e., 12.5 to 25 mg hydrochlorothiazide), although this side effect may have occurred with the earlier recommended initial dose (100 mg) that was employed in the first 14 multicenter trials. Moreover, the dose of hydrochlorothiazide employed was 100 mg (or more) per day. Since these studies were reported, the initial dose of that thiazide has been 12.5 to 25 mg with possible increase to the full dose of 50 mg per day. Nevertheless, alternative possibilities may be offered for the so-called lack of prevention of CHD. These deaths may have resulted from cardiac arrhythmias or other causes of sudden cardiac death which may have been related to hypokalemia (and/or hypomagnesemia) associated with the higher diuretic doses employed in those earlier trials. Thus, in subsequent analyses of multicenter studies (see reference to Thijs, et al, 1992) where in lower doses of thiazides were employed in elderly patients with hypertension, the reduction in stroke and coronary heart disease deaths were realized. The earlier predictions by Collins, et al were

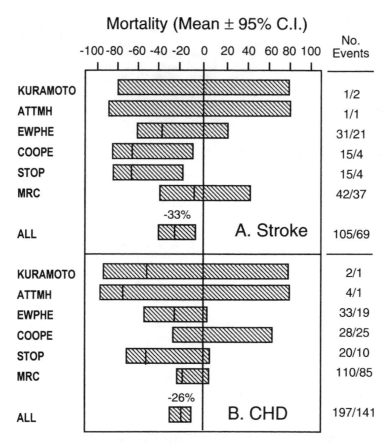

Figure 7.5. Meta-analysis coronary outcome effects of blood pressure reduction on stroke and CHD events in elderly patients. (Thijs, et al *J Hypertens,* 1992,10:1103–1109).

35 to 40 and 20 to 25 percent, respectively, for stroke and coronary heart disease, respectively, and these reductions reported by Thijs, et al were 33 and 26 percent respectively (Figure 7.5).

Although the following represents yet another investigator's line of thinking, I truly believe that the following concept is based upon sound pathophysiological principles. First, as indicated earlier in this monograph, hypertensive and epicardial occlusive atherosclerotic coronary heart diseases are two distinctly different disease processes, albeit they are closely interrelated and may certainly exacerbate one another. Myocardial infarction is the end point of atherosclerosis of the larger, epicardial coronary arteries, whereas hypertension is a disease of the smaller-resistance coronary (and other systemic) arterioles. The former disease results from lipid and plaque deposition in the coronary arterial intima that eventually obliterates the arterial lumina and fractures the plaque. In contrast, hypertensive coronary arteriolar disease (i.e., the underlying lesion of microvascular angina) is associated with: increased arterial pressure, total peripheral and coronary vascular resistances, aortic impedance, and left ventricular afterload; left ventricular hypertrophy; reduced coronary flow and flow reserve; altered blood viscosity; and increased myocardial oxygen demand. Thus, each of these two diseases follows its own protracted natural history over a lifetime, although, as suggested, each also complicates the other (Figure 7.2). Second, the earlier multicenter studies included in the meta-analysis primarily were involved with patients whose average age was 45 years (or more). Many were male and smoked. We know from autopsies of soldiers killed in the Korean and Vietnam Wars that atherosclerotic lesions were already present in these young (most 18 to 21 years) men. Third, most of these multicenter studies were double-blinded and placebo-controlled; their independent ethics monitoring committee terminated them prematurely when active drug treatment had been shown to protect the patients from stroke and other hypertension-related events. Myocardial infarction had not yet occurred with sufficient frequency to fulfill the meta-analytic statistical prediction of CHD.

Hypertensive-CHD Deaths

Following this line of pathophysiological reasoning, it seems highly reasonable to me that the deaths resulting from "coronary heart disease" could very well have included deaths from hypertensive just as well as from atherosclerotic coronary heart diseases. Both diseases may produce fatalities through similar clinical outcomes (e.g., arrhythmias, acute congestive heart failure, angina pectoris, sudden cardiac death), although the underlying pathophysiological mechanisms may have been founded on different bases (Figure 7.2). Thus, since the objectives of the early multicenter trials were to demonstrate safety and efficacy of antihypertensive therapy as well as prevention of hypertension-related events, the studies could hardly be faulted for "failure to prevent myocardial infarction." As suggested above, another explanation postulated for lack of protection from CHD may be that the diuretics may have induced electrolyte imbalance, which could have produced arrhythmias and sudden cardiac death. Most patients in these earlier multicenter trials had more severe disease and additional risk factors that may have been exacerbated by electrolyte imbalance, diminished contractile myocardial contractility, and coronary flow reserve that could be related to hypertensive coronary arteriolar disease and LVH. Indeed, this may very well have occurred in the Multiple Risk Factor Intervention Trial (MRFIT) in which one of the groups of (Stage I) patients did, in fact, have more abnormal ECGs than the usual care treatment group. That group did have more CHD deaths.

J-Shaped Curve Phenomenon

Another recent series of analyses has been related to the heart in hypertension. These reports concerned the relationship between deaths from myocardial infarction and pretreatment diastolic pressure levels and the extent to which diastolic pressure may be reduced by antihypertensive treatment. These analyses demonstrated a "J-shaped curve" phenomenon which suggested that those patients with lower pretreatment diastolic pressures (i.e., less than 85 mmHg) had a greater risk of death from myocardial infarction than those patients with higher diastolic pressures (85 to 89 mmHg). This risk increased further in those patients whose pretreatment diastolic pressures were 90 mmHg and more (Figure 7.6). Several conclusions derived from this analysis suggested, therefore, that patients with mildly elevated diastolic pressures should not be subjected to vigorous antihypertensive therapy. Support for the concept of the J-shaped curve phenomenon was offered by the pathophysiological knowledge that myocardial perfusion is dependent upon the diastolic pressure level. Although this J-curve phenomenon may or may not be real, its pathophysiological concept is

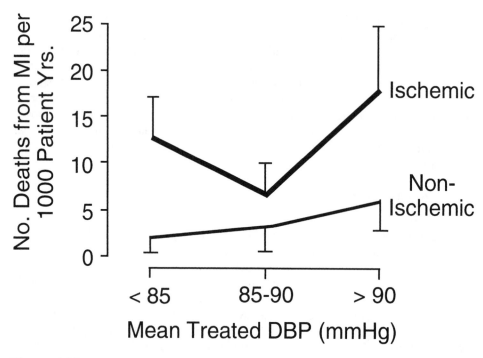

Figure 7.6. J-shaped curve phenomenon that was initially postulated by Cruick-shank et al. (*Lancet* 1987;1:581–584).

sound. However, it is also important to point out that the existence of a J-curve had not been demonstrated in several recent multicenter studies involving patients with diastolic or isolated systolic hypertension (e.g., SHEP, MRC, STOP-Hypertension) as well as other studies that have included primarily normotensive patients with severe atherosclerotic coronary artery disease. Each of these studies employed one of several commonly used antihypertensive agents (e.g., beta-adrenergic receptor inhibitors to prevent a second myocardial infarction; ACE inhibitors to prevent subsequent cardiac failure) following myocardial infarction or further morbidity (in patients with left ventricular dysfunction). In all of these reports, diastolic (and systolic) pressure was significantly reduced in all treated groups, and a J-curve phenomenon was neither detected nor reported. Actually, not only was cardiac failure significantly prevented, but ACE inhibition therapy also protected these severely ill patients from subsequent myocardial infarction and death. Nevertheless, at this time, it seems wise to recommend that arterial pressure should be reduced slowly and carefully, particularly in patients with LVH or with evidence of ischemic heart disease.

Symptomatic Coronary Insufficiency

As already indicated, insufficiency (i.e., inadequacy) of oxygen delivery to the hypertension-induced hypertrophied myocardium is produced by increased tension of the left ventricle. The two determinants of left ventricular tension are systolic pressure and the transverse diameter of the ventricular chamber itself. Both of these factors are increased in hypertensive LVH; and myocardial oxygen delivery capacity and flow reserve are also diminished in patients with hypertensive LVH. Thus, coronary insufficiency is inherent to hypertensive heart disease, and, more often than not, this is exacerbated by coexisting epicardial coronary arterial disease. The latter may be on the basis of coronary arterial spasm or by occlusive epicardial coronary arterial disease. In both of these arterial diseases, coronary blood flow may also be diminished by endothelial dysfunction which has been associated with impaired synthesis of one of the local coronary arterial vasodilators, nitric oxide. It is of interest (as suggested above) that this defect in endothelial generation of nitric oxide may be produced by hypertensive vascular disease and atherosclerosis, aging, and even habitual cigarette smoking. In any event, when coronary arterial disease is associated with hypertension, the goal of therapy should include reduced myocardial oxygen demand; this can be achieved by control of arterial pressure and reduction of left ventricular mass. In addition, improved myocardial perfusion (by calcium antagonists) and remodeling of the ventricular chamber, cardiac failure prophylaxis (with ACE inhibitors), and careful follow-up care to prevent hypokalemia and potential cardiac dysrhythmias are all wise therapeutic selections.

Beta-Adrenergic Receptor Blockers

These agents are also of great value in the hypertensive patient with LVH and coronary arterial insufficiency. The beta blockers have been shown to decrease left ventricular mass and wall thicknesses within three to four weeks in association with control of arterial pressure (Figure 7.7). Moreover, this is the one class of antihypertensive agents (exclusive of those compounds having intrinsic sympathomimetic activity) that

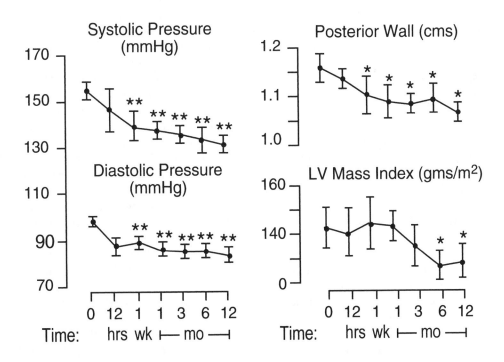

Figure 7.7. Time course regression of LVH with beta-adrenergic receptor blockade (Dunn FG: *Circulation* 1987;76:256–258).

has been shown, in controlled multicenter trials, to prevent a second myocardial infarction and death from cardiac arrhythmias. In fact, the beta-blocking agents have been particularly useful in patients with symptomatic coronary arterial insufficiency. Thus, by reducing arterial pressure and heart rate (i.e., the double product of systolic pressure and heart rate), the beta blockers are capable of reducing myocardial oxygen demand, thereby accounting for its beneficial effect in hypertensive (as well as normotensive) patients with angina pectoris. However, in those patients not demonstrating adequate improvement from angina pectoris with the beta blockers, the calcium antagonists have been demonstrated to be highly effective. This does not imply that the beta blocker needs to be discontinued; it may still prove to be of value in preventing a second myocardial infarction (should one have occurred). However, the physician should exercise particular care in prescribing a calcium antagonist together with a beta blocker since both agents may possess sufficient negative inotropic effect to predispose the patient to left ventricular decompensation.

Calcium Antagonists

In those patients with coronary arterial spasm, calcium antagonists not only provide control of arterial pressure but they may relieve the pain associated with that spasm or from occlusive epicardial disease. However, it is important to remember that these agents should be employed using their prolonged-acting formulations rather than with the short-duration action formulations (e.g., capsular formulation of nifedipine). Recent case study reports involving three short-acting formulations of calcium antagonists (i.e., nifedipine, diltiazem, and verapamil) suggested that those patients receiving one of these three calcium antagonists (i.e., the short-acting capsular formulation of nifedipine) had more myocardial infarction events than their control group of hypertensive patients, who did not receive calcium antagonists. One should keep in mind that a case study is a retrospective analysis and lacks the very real value of prospectively designed studies in which patients are assigned randomly to treatment and control groups. It should be recognized further that the authors of the case study indicated that their patients did not have cardiovascular disease. Obviously, they did since hypertension, per se, is a cardiovascular disease, many with LVH, many with impaired coronary flow and flow reserve, and many with endothelial dysfunction of the coronary arteries and arterioles. Moreover, most physicians are aware that it is reasonable to prescribe a calcium antagonist for the patient with more severe hypertension, particularly with LVH or angina pectoris. Nevertheless, it must be repeated that careful meta-analysis of studies conducted in hypertensive patients receiving the short-acting (capsular form of the calcium antagonist) nifedipine, unlike the other two agents (shorter-acting diltiazem or verapamil), may have provoked more coronary deaths. Indeed, subsequent analyses indicated that there were more myocardial infarction events in those patients who received the short-acting capsular formulation of nifedipine. Since the capsular formulation of nifedipine had never been approved for clinical use of patients with hypertension, this recommendation stands: Short-acting nifedipine should not be prescribed. Nevertheless, the calcium antagonist is a class of agents (the longer-acting agents, when appropriately used) that is of particular value for patients with spasm of the coronary arteries or with LVH associated with clinical evidence of coronary insufficiency (e.g., ST-segment changes with exercise testing or angina pectoris). Although the calcium antagonists have not been shown to prevent myocardial infarction in multicenter trials, one agent (i.e., diltiazem) has also been shown to protect the patient from a non-Q-wave infarction.

Angiotensin-Converting Enzyme Inhibitors.

Administration of these antihypertensive agents may also be highly effective in controlling arterial pressure and the associated increased oxygen demands of the hypertrophied left ventricle by reducing myocardial tension and by remodeling left ventricular architecture. As already indicated, an intrinsic or local renin-angiotensin system within the cardiac myocyte may be responsible (at least in part) for the reduction in left ventricular mass, although this may also be explained (perhaps, at least, in part) by increased kinins that also result from ACE inhibition. This enzyme that converts angiotensin I to angiotensin II is the same enzyme that inactivates bradykinin. In a series of independent multicenter, controlled trials over the past decade, most popularized by the first of these studies, the SAVE (Survival and Ventricular Enlargements Trial), not only have the ACE inhibitors been shown to prevent later development of congestive heart failure in the patient with a prior myocardial infarction, but this study also showed that the drug prevented a second myocardial infarction as well as death. Hence, in the patient with epicardial coronary arterial disease—particularly following myocardial infarction—the ACE inhibitors are particularly useful in controlling arterial pressure, preventing a second myocardial infarction and ensuing cardiac failure, and preventing premature death. Furthermore, the ACE inhibitors have been shown to be of particular value in counteracting the effects of defective nitric oxide production with endothelial disease. Ongoing studies are also in progress to determine the value of ACE inhibitors in preventing re-stenosis of bypassed coronary arteries or those vessels following angioplasty procedures. Other studies, involving the angiotensin II (type 1) receptor antagonist are in progress; preliminary reports have shown their efficacy in preventing cardiac failure (at least as well as the ACE inhibitor positive control group).

(Note: For specific details concerning each of the drugs comprising the foregoing classes of antihypertensive agents, their dosing, advice on side effects, and interactions, the reader is referred to the various specific tables in Chapter 5).

ANNOTATED BIBLIOGRAPHY

References selected to highlight those reports of studies that demonstrate the clinical progression of hypertensive heart disease

1. Frohlich ED, Tarazi RC, Dustan HP: Clinical-physiological correlations in the development of hypertensive heart disease. *Circulation* 1971;44:446–455.
2. Dunn FG, Chandraratna P, deCarvalho JGR, Basta LL, Frohlich ED: Pathophysiologic assessment of hypertensive heart disease with echocardiography. *Am J Cardiol* 1977;39:789–795.
3. Frohlich ED: Is reversal of left ventricular hypertrophy in hypertension beneficial? *Hypertension* 1991;18(I):133–138.
4. Frohlich ED: The first Irvine H. Page lecture: The mosaic of hypertension: Past, present, and future. *J Hypertens* 1988;6(Suppl 4):S2–S11.

5. Frohlich ED: Current Issues in Hypertension: Old Questions with New Answers and New Questions. *Med Clin North Am* 1992;76:1043–1056.
6. Frohlich ED: LVH, cardiac diseases and hypertension: Recent experiences. *J Am Coll Cardiol* 1989;14:1587–1594.
7. Frohlich ED, Apstein C, Chobanian AV, Devereux RB, Dustan HP, Dzau V, Fauad-Tarazi F, Horan MJ, Marcus M, Massie B, Pfeffer MA, Re RN, Roccella EJ, Savage D, Shub C: The heart in hypertension. *N Engl J Med* 1992;327:998–1008.
8. Sokolow M, Perloff D: Prognosis of essential hypertension treated conservatively. *Circulation* 1961;33:87–97.
9. Komuro I, Shibazaki Y, Kurabayashi M, Takaku F, Yazaki Y: Molecular cloning of gene sequences from rat heart rapidly responsive to pressure overload. *Circ Res* 1990;66:979–985.
10. Basan RS, Levy D: The role of hypertension in the pathogenesis of heart failure. A clinical mechanistic overview. *Arch Intern Med* 1996;156:1789–1796.
11. Frohlich ED: Pathophysiology of systemic arterial hypertension. In: *Hurst's The Heart,* 8th edition (Schlant RC, Alexander RW, O'Rourke RA, Roberts R, Sonnenblick EH, eds). McGraw-Hill, New York, 1993, pp. 1391–1401.
   Major reports dealing with the structural and functional characteristics of left ventricular hypertrophy
12. Meerson FZ: Compensatory hyperfunction, hyperadaptation, and insufficiency of the heart. In *The Failing Heart: Adaptation and Deadaptation* (Katz AM, ed). New York, Raven Press, 1983, pp. 47–66.
13. Grossman W, Jones D, McLaurin LP: Wall stress and patterns of hypertrophy in the human left ventricle. *J Clin Invest* 1975;56:56–64.
   Important echocardiographic studies that have led to the significance of LVH as a major cardiovascular risk factor
14. Levy D, Anderson KM, Savage DD, et al: Echocardiographically detected left ventricular hypertrophy: Prevalence and risk factors. The Framingham Heart Study. *Ann Intern Med* 1988;108:7–13.
15. Levy D, Garrison RJ, Savage DD, Kannel WB, Castelli WP: Prognostic implications of echocardiographically determined left ventricular mass in The Framingham Heart Study. *N Engl J Med* 1990;322:1561–1566.
16. Bikkina M, Levy D, Evans JC, Larson MG, Benjamin EJ, Wolf PA, Castelli WP: Left ventricular mass and the risk of stroke in an elderly cohort: The Framingham Heart Study. *JAMA* 1994;272:33–36.
17. Koren MJ, Devereux RB, Casale PN, Savage DD, Laragh JH: Relation of left ventricular mass and geometry to morbidity and mortality in uncomplicated essential hypertension. *Ann Intern Med* 1991;114:345–352.
18. Levy D, Salomon M, D'Agostino RB, Belanger AJ, Kannel WB: Prognostic implications of baseline electrocardiographic features and their serial changes in subjects with left ventricular hypertrophy. *Circulation* 1994;90:1786–1793.
19. Levy D, Larson MG, Vasan RS, Kannel WB, Ho KKL: The progression from hypertension to congestive heart failure. *JAMA* 1996;275:1557–1562.
20. Sheps S, Frohlich ED: Limited echocardiography for hypertensive left ventricular hypertrophy. *Hypertension* 1997;29:519–524.
   Reports that have suggested nonhemodynamic factors are important in the development and reversal of LVH

21. Frohlich ED, Tarazi RC: Is arterial pressure the sole factor responsible for hypertensive cardiac hypertrophy? *Am J Cardiol* 1979;44:959–963.
22. Tarazi RC, Frohlich ED: Is reversal of cardiac hypertrophy a desirable goal of antihypertensive therapy? *Circulation* 1987;75(I):113–117.
23. Frohlich ED: Is reversal of left ventricular hypertrophy in hypertension beneficial? *Hypertension* 1991;18(I):133–138.
    Reports emphasizing role of collagen and hormonal factors in development and reversal of LVH
24. Weber KT, Brilla CG: Pathological hypertrophy and cardiac interstitium. -Fibrosis and renin-angiotensin-aldosterone system. *Circulation.* 1991;83:1849–1865.
25. Morgan HE, Baker KM: Cardiac hypertrophy: mechanical, neural, and endocrine dependence. *Circulation* 1991;83:13–25.
26. Weber KT, Anverson P, Armstrong PW, Brilla CG, Burnett JC Jr. Cruickshank JM, Devereux RB, Giles TD, Korsgaardn, Leier CV, Mendelsohn FAO, Motz WH, Mulvany MJ, Strauer BE: Remodeling and reparation of the cardiovascular system. *J Am Coll Cardiol* 1992;20:3–16.
27. Weber KT, Sun Y, Guarda E: Structural remodeling in hypertensive heart disease and the role of hormones. *Hypertension* 1994;23(2):869–877.
28. Weber KT: Editorial. Monitoring tissue repair and fibrosis from a distance. *Circulation* 1997;96:2488–2492.
29. Arita M, Horinaka S, Frohlich ED: Biochemical components and myocardial performance after reversal of left ventricular hypertrophy in spontaneously hypertensive rats. *J Hypertens* 1993;11:951–959.
    Reports relating coronary flow in LVH and its reversal.
30. Marcus ML, Harrison DG, Chilian WM, et al: Alterations in the coronary circulation in hypertrophied ventricles. *Circulation* 1987;75(I):19–25.
31. Houghton JL, Frank MJ, Carr AA, et al: Relations among impaired coronary flow reserve, left ventricular hypertrophy and thallium perfusion defects in hypertensive patients without obstructive coronary artery disease. *J Am Coll Cardiol* 1990;15:43–51.
32. Scheler S, Wolfgang M, Strauer BE: Mechanisms of angina pectoris in patients with systemic hypertension and normal epicardial coronary arteries by arteriogram. *Am J Cardiol* 1994;73:478–482.
    Studies emphasizing importance of impaired endothelium-dependent vasodilation in patients with hypertension
33. Panza JA, Garcia CE, Kilcoyne CM, Quyyumi AA, Cannon RO III: Impaired endothelium-dependent vasodilation in patients with essential hypertension. Evidence that nitric oxide abnormality is not localized to a single signal transduction pathway. *Circulation* 1995;91:1732–1738.
34. Gerhard M, Roddy MA, Creager SJ, Creager MA: Aging progressively impairs endothelium-dependent vasodilation in forearm resistance vessels of humans. *Hypertension* 1996;27:849–853.
35. Treasure CB, Klein JC, Vita JA, Manoukianu SV, Renwixh GH, Selwyn AP, Ganz P, Alexander RW: Hypertension and left ventricular hypertrophy are associated with impaired endothelium-mediated relaxation in human coronary artery resistance vessels. *Circulation* 1993;87:86–93.
36. Frohlich ED: 1996 Arthur C. Corcoran Lecture: Influence of nitric oxide and angiotensin II on renal involvement in hypertension. *Hypertension* 1997;2:188–193.

Reports suggesting the participation of the J-shaped curve phenomenon in hypertension and myocardial infarction

37. Cruickshank JM, Thorp JM, Zacharias FJ: Benefits and potential harm of lowering high blood pressure. *Lancet* 1987;1:581–584.
38. Cruickshank JM: Coronary flow reserve and the J-curve relation between diastolic blood pressure and myocardial infarction. *BMJ* 1988;297:1227–1230.
39. Collins C, Peto R. MacMahon S. Hebert H, Hebach NH, Eberlein KA, Godwin J, Olzilbash N, Taylor JO, Hennekens CH: Blood pressure, stroke and coronary heart disease. Part 2. Short-term reductions in blood pressure overview of randomised drug trials in their epidemiological context. *Lancet* 1990;335:827–838.
40. Thijs L, Fagard R, Lijnen P, Staessen J, VanHoot R, Amery A: A meta-analysis of outcome trials in elderly hypertensives. *J Hypertens* 1992;10:1103–1109.
41. MacMahon S, Peto R, Cutler J, Collins R, Sorlie P, Neaton J, Abbott R, Godwin J, Dyer A, Stamler J: Blood pressure, stroke, and coronary heart disease. Part I. Prolonged differences in blood pressure: Prospective observational studies corrected for the regression dilution bias. *Lancet* 1990;335:765–774.

Chapter 8

The Hypertensive Patient with Renal Arterial Disease and with Renal Involvement in Hypertension

RENAL ARTERIAL DISEASE

General

Several general considerations are worth stating before we consider the clinical problem of hypertension resulting from renal arterial disease. First, renal arterial lesions are found in normotensive as well as hypertensive individuals, especially if these patients have coexisting atherosclerosis. Thus, atherosclerotic renal arterial lesions are not infrequently observed in normotensive patients undergoing renal arteriography for a comprehensive assessment of atherosclerotic occlusive disease involving other organs. This point is worth considering as we now find an increased frequency of the performance of a renal arteriogram after a patient undergoes a more complete coronary arteriographic study. Second, renal arterial disease is frequently said to be a rare primary cause of systemic arterial hypertension. Actually, several reports have indicated that renal arterial disease (i.e., renovascular hypertension) may be the primary cause of hypertension in three to five percent of patients with hypertension. This means that using the presently conservative estimation of hypertension in the United States, upwards of 1.5 to 2.5 million patients with hypertension may have renal arterial disease as a primary causation of the disease. And, as a third point of importance, renal arterial disease may complicate the course of patients with essential hypertension, especially in those older people whose hypertension has become more difficult to manage because of the development of an occlusive atherosclerotic renal arterial lesion.

Pathophysiology

As suggested above, both normotensive and hypertensive patients may have renal arterial disease, but the disease only becomes clinically significant when the arterial lesion sufficiently compromises the renal and intrarenal hemodynamics sufficiently enough to stimulate the renopressor system. At that point when the renal hemodynamics are sufficiently compromised, the renal ischemia stimulates an increased release of renin by the juxtaglomerular cells which, in turn, promotes an increased generation of angiotensin II.

The increase in circulating plasma renin activity and generated angiotensin II raises arterial pressure through two predominant mechanisms: (1) arteriolar constriction that increases total peripheral resistance and, hence, the arterial pressure and (2) by secondarily promoting a release of aldosterone from the adrenal cortex which, in turn, produces specific metabolic changes. The secondary hyperaldosteronism thus produced is manifested by hypokalemic alkalosis which is associated with increased plasma renin activity, increased circulating aldosterone level and urinary secretion, and sodium retention. The generated angiotensin II also has additional hypertension favoring actions, including stimulation of adrenal medullary release of catecholamines; interaction with norepinephrine in medullary brain centers and at the peripheral nerve ending to augment adrenergic outflow; stimulation of thirst centers in the brain; and stimulation of local autocrine/paracrine factors that modulate arterial pressure and blood flow as well as that promote protein synthesis in cardiac and arteriolar myocytes. In patients with unilateral renal arterial disease and hypertension, the plasma volume will contract in proportion to the height of diastolic pressure and the increased total peripheral resistance. In addition to the foregoing physiological consequences of stimulating renin release by an ischemic kidney with ensuing generation of angiotensin II, other pathophysiological effects may also result, including interaction with catecholamines and vasopressin; possible stimulation of local renin angiotensin systems (e.g., in heart, arteries, brain, and elsewhere); and, of course, promotion of mitogenic structural changes in the heart, arterioles, and kidneys.

Experience has taught us that when blood is sampled from the renal veins, a ratio of plasma renin activity in the vein from the affected kidney of 1.6 and greater than the unaffected kidney predicts humoral as well as hemodynamic significance of the unilateral renal arterial lesion. Such evaluation of bilateral renal arterial disease is less clear-cut.

Diagnosis

Clearly the patient's clinical history is of value with this, the most common of the secondary forms of hypertension (excluding the over-the-counter and street-drug-associated forms of secondary hypertension). Among the more pertinent historical features of renal arterial disease are the negative family history of hypertension; the onset of uncontrollable hypertension in a hypertensive patient whose pressure elevation was well controlled; hypertension associated with inappropriately impaired renal function; the finding of upper abdominal or flank bruits (particularly those audible in diastole as well as systole); precipitation of severe accelerated or malignant hypertension; and the appearance of hypertension in children, particularly those without a family history of hypertension (Table 8.1).

A large number of screening laboratory tests are now available for the diagnosis of significant renal arterial disease, all with varying sensitivity and specificity (Table 8.2). Nevertheless, the "gold standard" for the clinical diagnosis (in my opinion) still remains with the selective renal arteriogram since it confirms the presence of disease and the extent of involvement of the renal arteries and is an excellent means for hemodynamic, anatomical, and natural history assessment. The clinician should also realize that the size (i.e., length) of the kidney is an excellent tip-off for the degree of significance since a smaller kidney suggests significant arterial occlusive disease (although unilateral renal atrophy should always be kept in mind). In this respect, one should remember that the left kidney is normally 0.5 cm longer than the right; thus, a 1.0- to 1.5-cm difference should stimulate suspicion. Delay of appearance of radiographic contrast material on intravenous urography with hyperconcentration and delay of disappearance should also provoke some suspicion. Radioactive renography may also be helpful with a delayed appearance and disappearance of the tagged radionuclide is also of importance. A base-

Table 8.1. Clinical Clues Suggesting Renovascular Hypertension

Severe hypertension in a young child, young adult, or adult more than 50 years old.

Sudden development of or worsening of preexisting hypertension at any age.

Systolic/diastolic upper abdominal or flank bruit.

Hypertension associated with unexplained impairment of renal function (suggests significant bilateral renal arterial disease).

Impairment of renal function in response to angiotensin converting enzyme inhibitor therapy (suggests bilateral disease).

Sudden worsening of renal function in hypertensive patient.

Hypertension refractory to appropriate three-drug regimen.

Development of accelerated or malignant hypertension.

Unilateral small kidney discovered by any clinical study.

Extensive occlusive atherosclerotic disease of the coronary, cerebral, or peripheral circulation.

line renogram study may be of value since it will provide the clinician with a measurable index of blood flow and renal viability should postoperative complications arise (including possible occlusion of the renal artery). In this regard, preoperative isotopic renography (with renal flow and scan) are very useful procedures; and, in recent years, this has been enhanced with studies before and then after administration of the more rapid acting angiotensin-converting enzyme (ACE) inhibitor captopril (Table 8.2). Finally, measurement of peripheral plasma renin activity (along with indexing to daily sodium intake) is also of value. This assay is enhanced much for diagnosis of renal arterial disease with the measurement of bilateral renal venous plasma renin activity measurements. Thus, a ratio of 1.6 favoring the affected kidney (affected to unaffected kidneys) strongly supports a physiologically significant unilateral renal arterial lesion.

Types of Arterial Lesions and Management

The type of renal arterial lesion pathologically has an important bearing on the natural history of the disease. Identification of the renal arterial lesion arteriographically should be of great value in defining these lesions. Therefore, it goes without saying that much can be learned by a clear selective arteriogram; this requires proper and appropriate positioning of the patient to permit adequate detail of the lesions. This is particularly important with orificial lesions.

The severity of the hypertensive disease is, in part, related to the severity of the hemodynamic effects of the renal arterial lesion, the secondary ischemia, the amount of plasma renin activity that is released by the affected kidney, and, clearly, the amount of angiotensin II that is generated. However, in addition, the severity of the hypertension is also related to whether there was preexisting hypertension, coexisting diseases, and, of course, preexisting renal parenchymal function. Clearly, if there is total (i.e., absolute) occlusion of the renal artery by the lesion, autonephrectomy may result with an ensuing actual "cure" of the previously normotensive patient from the renal arterial disease.

If the renal arterial disease is unilateral, treatment of the patient with an ACE inhibitor will inhibit the amount of angiotensin II that will be generated and, therefore, will reduce the level of the arterial pressure elevation. However, if the patient happens to have bilateral occlusive disease of the renal arteries, both kidneys will become ischemic and will release increased amounts of renin. As a result, renal function may become impaired bi-

Table 8.2. Screening Tests for Renal Arterial Disease

Test	Findings in patients with renal arterial disease	Comments
Intravenous urography	>1.0 to 1.5-cm disparity in renal lengths Delayed appearance of dye Delayed excretion of dye	Low Sensitivity
Isotopic renography	Abnormalities in perfusion in stenotic kidney	Better sensitivity and specificity than intravenous urography
Plasma renin activity	Plasma renin activity increased	Medium sensitivity and specificity Low plasma renin activity makes renal arterial disease improbable Influenced by many conditions
Plasma renin activity with captopril	Hyperreninemia Plasma renin activity augmented	Better sensitivity and specificity than plasma renin activity alone Strict diagnostic criteria Poor discrimination of unilateral or bilateral renal arterial disease
Bilateral renal venous renin	Renin higher in stenotic (affected) side	Evaluate renal venous activity ratio ($\geq$ 1.6)
Duplex Doppler of renal arteries	Lower peak systolic velocity	Technical limitations with obesity or intestinal gas Only proximal lesions
Selective renal arteriography	Anatomic localization Collateral circulation Pathological lesion assessment	Stenosis does not mean renal ischemia 75% stenosis is highly significant Renal protection is advised with atheroma

laterally, renal failure may result, and a greater volume dependency of the hypertension will also result. Moreover, if the renal arterial disease is bilateral and an ACE is administered, there is less compensatory intrarenal changes and further aggravation of the hypertension with possible impairment of renal function; in fact, malignant hypertension may even result.

As indicated above, therefore, much can be learned by performing selective renal arteriography. First, it gives the physician a clear idea as to the degree and significance of the arterial disease. It also provides an excellent prognostic concept as to the natural history disease since a number of prospective and retrospective studies have provided an important concept for pathologic–radiologic correlation of the lesion, its potential complications, and an enlightened means for a more immediate and long-term management of the disease. In general, arterial lesions are of two types, atherosclerotic and nonatherosclerotic (or fibrosing).

Atherosclerotic Lesions   These lesions are usually orificial in location and are at the proximal one-third of the main renal artery. The selective arteriogram will usually demonstrate eccentricity of the occlusive lesion, because the atherosclerotic plaque is located on one wall of the vessel or the lesion may be associated poststenotic dilation of the renal artery having a "boggy" or balloon-like appearance (Figure 8.1). Atherosclerotic lesions are more common in men, particularly if the patient is younger than 45 years of age. If the patient is older, the lesion frequently may be bilateral; and the atherosclerosis may be a diffuse vascular disease. Because of this potential, before surgical repair of the lesion is considered, the patient should be fully evaluated for coexistent atherosclerotic occlusive disease involving the coronary, carotid, splanchnic, and peripheral arteries as well as the aorta. Awareness of these possibilities should prepare the physician for potential problems before and during surgical intervention is considered and should help to obviate unanticipated complications. Furthermore, if surgical intervention is considered, repair should take into consideration not only the presence of an occlusive arterial lesion, but the purpose for which the operature procedure is being considered: surgical remission of the hypertensive disease; improved control of arterial pressure even if drug therapy will still be necessary; preservation of existing renal function; or management of the secondary problems of the arterial disease (e.g., dissection of the renal artery, rupture and repair of arterial bleeding, or thrombosis of a branch of the artery associated with severe pain and dissection).

Nonatherosclerotic Lesions   The fibrosing diseases of the renal artery are associated with different natural histories; and each of the lesions seems to have a different natural history of disease. Fortunately, the fibrosing lesions have very different radiographic appearances of the arterial lesion; this depends upon the involved layer(s) of the arterial wall. Credit for our understanding of these lesions, their natural history, complications, and management must be given to the teams of radiologists, pathologists, surgeons, and clinicians at the Cleveland and Mayo Clinics in the late 1960s and early 1970s. They are responsible for elucidating the fascinating and important correlations between the arteriographic, pathological, and clinical characteristics of the lesions. In those days it was frequently the practice to resect the lesion, to effect reconstitution of the artery and, then, to study the resected lesion pathologically.

Perhaps the most common of the fibrosing lesions of the renal artery is that of *medial* (or perimedial) *fibroplasia*. This disease is not infrequently bilateral, occurs more commonly in younger women, and, on arteriography, has the classical appearance

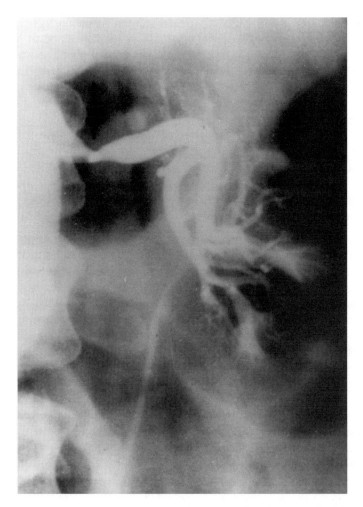

Figure 8.1.   Atherosclerotic lesion appearing smooth and eccentric (arrow) with poststenotic dilation. This lesion is proximal in the main renal artery, often comprising the ostium. The distal renal artery and its branches appear normal. The lesion may also appear with poststenotic dilation or "bogginess."

of the so-called "string of beads" lesion (Figure 8.2). This lesion appears as multifocal sequential areas of fibrosis within the media of the arterial wall that do not disrupt the external limiting membrane of the media. The disease disrupts the internal elastic membrane, thereby giving the arteriographic appearance of the "string of beads." The disease, fortunately, progresses slowly and may be rarely complicated by dissection or thrombosis. Its rate of progression is slower than that of atherosclerotic lesions or some of the other fibrosing lesions. Hence, this lesion may be managed with antihypertensive therapy that can be selected to inhibit the renin-angiotensin system [e.g., ACE inhibitors, angiotensin II (type 1) receptor antagonists, or even the beta-adrenergic receptor or other adrenergic inhibitors]. It is important, however, to point out that the ACE inhibitors should not be prescribed if the renal arterial disease is bilateral or if there is unilateral renal arterial disease in a patient with unilateral renal arterial disease in a solitary kidney (see discussion above). Alterna-

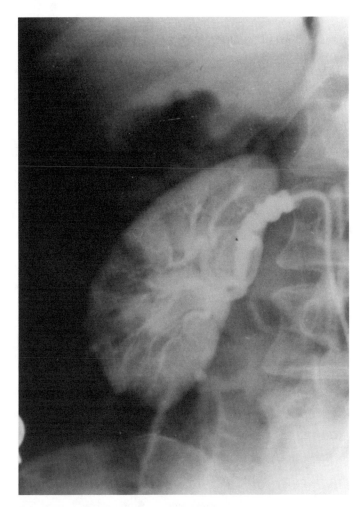

Figure 8.2. Medial fibroplasia: "String of beads" aspect of the lesion is explained by multiple and confluent aneurysmal formations. This lesion is not severely stenosing, and it is depicted as in this arteriogram affecting the midrenal artery. The primary branches appear normal in this patient.

tively, the lesion may be corrected by percutaneous renal arterial angioplasty. However, before this is begun, the physician must bear in mind that the lesion is frequently found in the contralateral kidney; if it is not found at the time of the initial renal arteriogram, then it may be detected at some later time when the lesion may appear. This is an important consideration, particularly if surgical repair or nephrectomy is considered (or becomes necessary) since this will leave the patient with a solitary kidney if, at that later time, disease then appears in the contralateral renal artery. Following this same line of thinking, it is particularly appropriate to be certain that multiple radiographic views of the renal artery be obtained in order to be clearly certain as to the presence, extent, and involvement of the entire renal artery and its branches. This is of importance not only in patients with atherosclerotic renal arterial lesions in which the extent, and shape of the orificial lesions must be clear, but also in those arteries with fibrosing lesions. The latter lesions appear in the proximal or mid-third of the renal artery, and they may be identified without certainty as to whether there are lesions in the distal third of the artery or even in the more distal secondary and tertiary branchings of the artery.

The two remaining renal arterial lesions may be more severely stenosing. In contrast to the intramural location of medial fibroplastic disease are the hyperplastic lesions of *intimal fibroplasia* (Figure 8.3) and of subadventitial fibroplasia (Figure 8.4). The former intimal lesion, like the atherosclerotic lesions, is frequently in the proximal third of the renal artery (although it may occur more distally), and is characterized by a circumferential proliferation of fibrous tissue within the intima of the vessel wall. On arteriography, the lesion has a more symmetrical appearance of the stenosis which produces a more severe physiological impairment of the vascular hemodynamics. Although this lesion often occurs in the proximal third of the renal artery, it may also occur more distally and, not infrequently, into the branches of

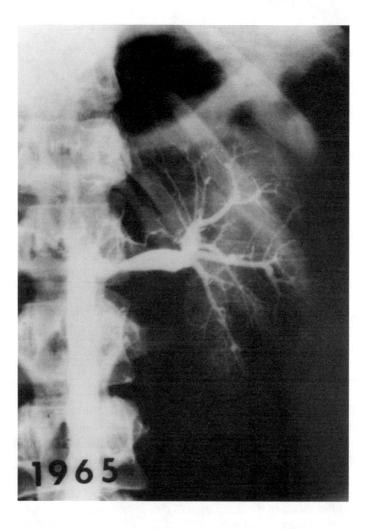

Figure 8.3.   Intimal fibroplasia: The intimal proliferation of fibrous disease produce a smooth, generally more symmetric and highly stenosing lesion.

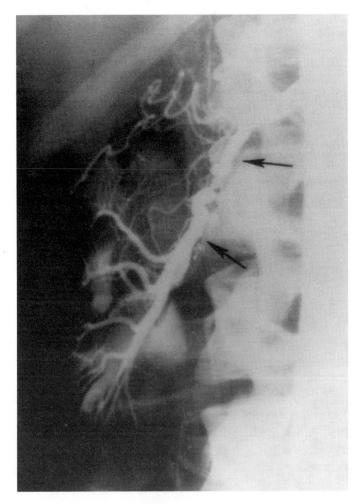

Figure 8.4.   Subadventitial fibroplasia. A severely stenosing lesion with radiologic appearance of aneurysms that are less confluent than those of medial fibroplasia. Here the aneurysmal dissection reflects disruption of the external limiting membrane. Note the characteristic collateral flow surrounding the artery (arrows) and the upper part of the kidney, indicating considerable renal ischemia.

the main renal artery. These lesions occur in children as well as in adults, and there does not seem to be a gender preference. The lesion of intimal fibroplasia severely restricts the lumen of the artery; this is complicated by severely elevated arterial pressures and arterial complications including dissection, rupture with hemorrhage, and thrombosis (Figure 8.5). The lesions of *subadventitial fibroplasia* appear arteriographically as more severe stenosis, and the fibrous disease frequently invades the external elastic membrane to involve the subadventitial area of the arterial wall with fibrous tissue. The disease can produce a variety of luminal irregularities with the development of collateral vessels on the arteriogram. These lesions frequently progress even to involve both kidneys, and the disease may be associated with dissection and hemorrhage. As a result, although pharmacological

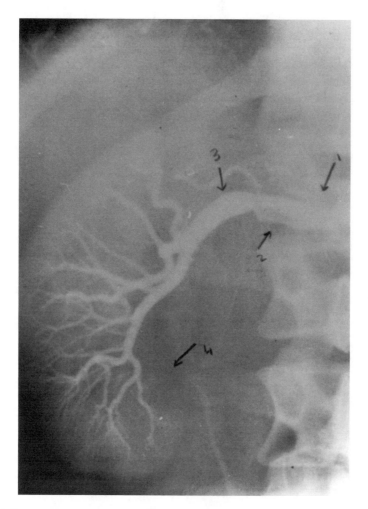

Figure 8.5.   Complications of intimal fibroplasia. In this selective renal arteriogram, the intimal dissection has occurred, and a double lumen is observed before
the stenosing presence of collateral vessels.

therapy is frequently useful, the clinician should consider early and periodic surgical consultation with repeated selective arteriographic studies if surgical or angio-
plastic treatment is not pursued.

Treatment

As already indicated, the definitive diagnosis of renovascular hypertension is firmly
established by the demonstration of the arterial lesion(s) with renal arteriography. The
treatment of the arterial disease, however, is not nearly as clear cut. In general, selection of the mode of treatment is based upon the overall medical condition of the
patient; risks and side effects of the therapeutic modality; past experience with treatment of the patient; patho-radiographic type of arterial lesion; and availability of ex-

perienced radiographers (for diagnosis as well as percutaneous transluminal renal angioplasty (PTRA or PTCA) and surgeons.

Medical Treatment   The pharmacological management of hypertension resulting from renal arterial disease has remarkably improved in recent years as it has been possible to select those drugs that are more specific in suppressing renopressor mechanisms. In the earlier years of antihypertensive drug therapy, hypertension secondary to a renal arterial disease could be controlled with the available drugs albeit less specifically and, usually, with more side effects. Since the release of renin from the kidney could be suppressed by adrenergic inhibiting drugs and beta-blocking agents, these modalities were the most effective at that time. However, these drugs usually required the addition of diuretics which complicated further the secondary hyperaldosteronism related to the renal arterial disease. Of course, the exacerbated hyperkalemic alkalosis could be ameliorated by spironolactone or potassium supplements; but, these approaches were dramatically improved with the advent of the angiotensin converting enzyme (ACE) inhibitors and, more recently, with the angiotensin II (type 1) receptor inhibitors (AII antagonists). Of course, even these agents may provide suboptimal control of pressure, and, in these cases, the addition of a thiazide diuretic will add to the overall effectiveness of medical management. A potassium-sparing diuretic agent may be used, but under these clinical circumstances, the physician should carefully follow serum electrolyte levels (especially potassium) since the ACE inhibitor or AII antagonists may predispose the patient to severe hyperkalemia because of the inhibition of the renopressor system. (The reader is referred to chapters 4 and 5 for further discussion of medical therapy, clinical pharmacology, and indications for specific therapy.)

Special word of caution must be added to the selection of pharmacological therapy since, even though arterial pressure may be well controlled, the vascular disease may progress. This progression of the occlusive atherosclerotic or nonatherosclerotic lesion may be manifested by: further elevation of arterial pressure requiring more intensive drug therapy; more severe occlusion of the renal arterial lesion; thrombosis; dissection; hemorrhage; and progressive impairment of renal function. It goes without saying, a comprehensive medical treatment in these patients should include vigorous hypolipidemic therapy, weight control, exercise, and cessation of tobacco consumption. Furthermore, it is extremely important to follow renal function carefully as well as the patient's history for symptoms of pain and hematuria and loss of blood pressure control. These complications can occur within the ipsilateral renal artery as well as in the contralateral artery. Progressive occlusion of the atherosclerotic lesion may occur in as much as half (or more) of patients and is more likely in those lesions with greater occlusive disease. In some patients developing total occlusion of the artery, there may be no associated symptoms, and blood pressure may actually normalize as a consequence of the "autonephrectomy."

As suggested by the foregoing discussion of the types of fibrosing lesions involving the renal arteries, prediction of progression or complications of the arterial disease may be related to the nature of the lesion(s). Some of these lesions are more likely to be encountered later bilaterally (e.g., medial fibroplasia) and others may, more frequently, be complicated by thrombosis, dissection, or hemorrhage.

Angioplasty   PTRA, (percutaneous transluminal renal angioplasty), while not fully medical therapy, is not surgical. Its efficacy is best in more experienced hands and when careful radiographic demonstration of the patient lesions is made. Thus, an orificial lesion is not infrequently difficult to demonstrate or assess if only an anteroposterior projection of the arteriographic lesion is made. Moreover, these orificial lesions are less successfully approached by PTRA than those other lesions that may be demonstrable in the proximal third of the main renal artery (possibly due to the difficulty in demonstrating most completely the extent of the luminal occlusion of the lesion by a single radiographic projection). It follows that patients with bilaterally occlusive atherosclerotic renal vascular disease will have a lesser success rate from PTRA than in patients with unilateral disease. Success rate for PTRA has been best in those patients with fibrosing renal arterial lesions (Table 8.3). Particular care must also be made in those patients having larger aneurysmal disease. In more recent years, placement of intra-arterial stents has been pursued, but experience with this approach is too recent to express success and restenosis rates.

Complications from these forms of catheter treatment obviously varies with the experience of the angiographer. These vary from hematoma at the puncture site, renal arterial spasm (which may be reversed with nitroglycerine), intravascular thrombosis, embolization (not only from the arterial plaque but from preexisting thrombi), vessel rupture, and impairment of renal function as a result of nephrotoxicity from the radiographic contrast material.

Surgery Choice of the surgical procedure also varies with the form of disease and experience of the surgeon. If there is no evidence of circulation of blood flow to the affected kidney by arteriography and/or by radioisotopic scanning) there may be no need for nephrectomy; autonephrectomy may result. However, if the involved kidney is very small and atrophic, nephrectomy may be the most reasonable choice of surgery. Surgical treatment may be expected to be most successful in those patients with fibrosing renal arterial lesion—either those in whom PTRA was not feasible or if restenosis has appeared. In those patients in whom revascularization is deemed necessary, complete bypass of the arterial lesion(s) is performed. Under these circumstances, in my experience, selection for such treatment in patients with atherosclerotic disease should be pursued: when control of arterial pressure has not been possible with medical therapy or PTRA; in order to prevent further progression of disease; or to preserve progressive deterioration in renal function when there is bilateral renal arterial disease. In the latter group of patients with bilateral atherosclerotic disease, surgical revascularization at present seems to be more effective than PTRA.

Table 8.3. Relative Efficacy of Revascularization Versus Percutaneous Transluminal Renal Angioplasty for Renal Arterial Disease[a]

Lesion	Success with PTRA[b] (%)	Success with Revascularization (%)
Atherosclerotic		
Nonostial (20%)	80–90	90
Ostial (80%)	25–30	90
Fibrosing lesions		
Main renal artery (50%)	80–90	90
Branch (50%)	—	90

[a] From Pohl MA: Renovascular hypertension: An internist's point of view. In (Punzi H, Flamembaum W, eds): *Hypertension.* New York, Futura Publishing Co, 1989, p 367 (with permission).
[b] PTRA, percutaneous transluminal renal angioplasty.

NEPHROSCLEROSIS AND END-STAGE RENAL DISEASE

General

In contrast to the very satisfying reports concerning the beneficial effects of long-term antihypertensive therapy in preventing and reducing morbidity and mortality from stroke and coronary heart disease in patients with essential hypertension, the experience with end-stage renal disease (ESRD) is just the opposite. Over these past several decades there has been an unrelenting increase in the numbers of patients with hypertension with progressive loss of renal function and parenchymal renal involvement by hypertensive vascular disease (i.e., nephrosclerosis). This has resulted in increasing numbers of patients who have developed ESRD resulting in death or requiring long-term dialysis. Thus, until recently it does not seem to have been possible to prevent the progression of renal involvement from hypertension from progressing with standard antihypertensive therapy. However, it has been possible to manage the renal failure with long-term hemodialysis or with peritoneal dialysis; and, more recently, renal failure has been effectively reversed by renal transplantation (even in patients with only essential hypertension). This is not to say that every patient who progressed into ESRD had renal involvement from severe (essential) hypertensive nephrosclerosis. However, by far, the vast majority of those patients with essential hypertension that has progressed from milder degrees of proteinuria to unrelenting loss of renal excretory function has been hypertensive patients who were either black or who had coexisting diabetes mellitus (Figure 8.6).

The Paradox

Nephrologists have been perplexed by this seeming paradox. Thus, on one hand, long-term antihypertensive drug therapy has been able to reduce morbidity and mortality from stroke and coronary heart disease and, on the other hand, this therapy has not been able to have similar results with renal involvement. Although at the present time this problem remains unresolved and is the subject of intense study, several explanations have been offered. First, renal involvement from hypertensive vascular disease may not be responsive or reversible to antihypertensive therapy. A second possibility is that the goal antihypertensive treatment pressures of the past (diastolic pressures less than 90 mmHg) were not optimal and that the goal diastolic pressures in the future must be much lower (e.g., perhaps 70 or 75 mmHg). An equally plausible possibility is a third possibility that the antihypertensive drug classes that have been used by the earlier long-term, controlled clinical trials may have been specific enough to affect target organ involvement in brain and heart, but it was not effective on the kidney. The following discussion presents the hemodynamic mechanisms concerned with the progression of hypertensive renal disease and how specific antihypertensive drugs may affect the progression of renal involvement in hypertension. Recent reports have indicated effectiveness of certain antihypertensive agents on diabetic renal disease; but no study, thus far, has been reported for patients with hypertensive renal disease.

Normal Renal and Glomerular Dynamics

Maintenance of normal renal excretory function is based on the assumption that renal blood flow is maintained normal and that it is associated with normal glomerular hemodynamics due to a fine hemodynamic balance between pre- and postglomerular arteriolar resistance. Inherent in this latter assumption is that the afferent

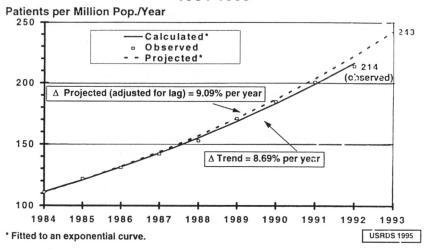

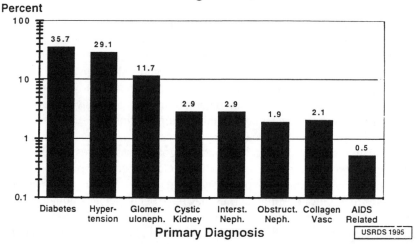

Figure 8.6. Progressive increase in end-stage renal disease in the United States from 1984 through 1993 (upper). The greatest number of these patients had diabetes or hypertension (lower). (From U.S. Renal Data System: USRDS 1995 Annual Data Report. The National Institutes of Health, National Institute of Diabetes and Digestive and Kidney Diseases, Bethesda MD, 1995. III. Incidence and causes of treated ESRD. *Am J Kidney Dis* 1995;26(Suppl 2):38–50.)

glomerular arterioles are able to dilate or constrict in response to changes in renal blood flow and thus regulate glomerular hydrostatic pressure from renal blood flow alterations. Moreover, the efferent glomerular arteriolar resistance is likewise able to respond to the myriad of factors that can alter its vascular smooth muscle tone so that the glomerular hydrostatic pressure can also ensure adequate glomerular filtration rate and urinary output. A number of hormonal, humoral, and neural factors participate in this exquisite regulation of glomerular dynamics in addition to the kidney's own autoregulatory ability of adjusting vascular resistance to changes in blood flow. (The reader is referred to Chapter 1 for further discussion.)

From a clinical point of view, it is difficult to assess changes in the glomerular dynamics, although it is possible to estimate these changes grossly. This can be done by measuring renal blood flow and glomerular filtration rate using the classical clearance methods of para-aminohippurate and inulin (or any of the other physiological and clinical surrogates including the serum creatinine concentration). The ratio of glomerular filtration rate to the renal blood flow is the renal filtration fraction; this index is of clinical value in obtaining some idea of the changing glomerular hydrostatic pressure. Thus, an increased renal filtration fraction may reflect increased glomerular hydrostatic pressure, ultrafiltration, protein excess in the mesangium, and glomerulosclerosis. Clinically, this assessment takes into consideration the average of all of the glomerulae that participate in overall renal function.

It is possible experimentally, however, to obtain a much clearer assessment of glomerular dynamic changes in response to disease or treatment by performing carefully controlled renal micropuncture studies. This technique, however, requires prolonged anesthesia, and the placement of a perfused kidney in a bath of controlled temperature while single-nephron hemodynamic clearance methods and tubular and capillary micropuncture measurements are obtained. In reality, it has been possible (through these techniques) to achieve a rather meaningful understanding of the pathophysiology of renal disease and the effects of antihypertensive therapy.

Experimental Hypertensive ESRD

To accomplish this overall assessment, a number of experimental models of hypertensive renal disease have been developed in recent years. In general, they generally have involved induction of renal failure by unilateral nephrectomy (usually with extirpation of some of the contralateral renal tissue) with or without the superimposition of additional factors (e.g., salt-loading, steroid administration, renal infarction, administration of other nephrotoxic agents or chemicals). To my way of thinking, none of these interventions are analogous to the patient with essential hypertension and the natural development of ESRD that progresses without surgical intervention that can transpire over many years.

Experiences with the SHR   More recently, we have been able to follow up on our earlier studies which suggested that naturally occurring ESRD occurs in the spontaneously hypertensive rat (SHR) with naturally developing genetic hypertension. Those studies have indicated that massive proteinuria with histological evidence of severe nephrosclerosis will develop if the SHR is followed until it is about one year of age. (The lifespan of a normotensive rat is about three years, and that of the SHR is no more than two years.) Hence, severe hypertensive nephrosclerosis can develop naturally in the SHR.

For this reason, we studied the 73-week-old male SHR (purchased at 21 weeks of age and followed carefully for the ensuing 52 weeks) and found that ESRD resulted and was, in fact, associated with pathological evidence of severe nephrosclerosis, marked proteinuria, and severely impaired renal micropuncture findings which indicated that the foregoing hemodynamic alterations do, in fact, favor glomerulosclerosis with ESRD. These micropuncture findings revealed severely reduced renal blood flow and glomerular filtration rate; increased afferent and efferent glomerular arteriolar resistance; and increased glomerular hydrostatic pressure. And, most interestingly, when these rats were treated with an ACE inhibitor, each of these pathophysiological alterations were reversed (if not normalized) within a three-week period of treatment.

Endothelial Dysfunction   Having demonstrated that the SHR can naturally develop ESRD with aging, we then developed a model of this naturally developing ESRD by administering (for three weeks) the nitric oxide synthase inhibitor N^ω-nitro-L-arginine methyl ester (L-NAME). We indicated in Chapter 7 that L-NAME inhibits local production of nitric oxide in the endothelium of blood vessels and that this experimentally induced alteration is very similar to the reduced endothelial production of nitric oxide that occurs with aging, hypertension, and atherosclerosis. We therefore administered the L-NAME for three weeks to 16- to 20-week-old SHRs and actually reproduced the very same ESRD with nephrosclerosis and the associated proteinuria and renal and glomerular dynamic alterations that we had just observed with aging in the SHR. Not only was ESRD produced within three weeks in these much younger SHR, but we were able to prevent this ESRD with the very same ACE inhibitor that we employed in the 73-week-old SHR. Moreover, we also reversed these very same alterations by administering that same ACE inhibitor for three weeks after the L-NAME had been given. Furthermore, not only was it possible to prevent and reverse ESRD in these L-NAME/SHR with ACE inhibitors, but we also were able to reverse these very same changes in 85-week-old SHRs (but without the necessity of giving L-NAME) by administering the amino acid precursor (L-arginine) for nitric oxide synthesis over three weeks to these rats.

Finally, we administered hydrochlorothiazide to the younger (20-week-old) L-NAME/SHR for three weeks and significantly exacerbated the same ESRD pathologically, hemodynamically, and clinically that we observed in the old SHRs and younger rats with L-NAME. Our studies in this area continue; but from these studies we may arrive at several tentative conclusions that have particular clinical relevance for patients with essential hypertension. First, ESRD can be demonstrated in naturally occurring hypertension by aging. Second, it is not valid to conclude that this renal target organ involvement in hypertension is not necessarily amenable to prevention or reversal with conventional antihypertensive therapy. Third, while the antihypertensive therapy that was used did, in fact, reduce arterial pressure, it was not necessary to reduce diastolic pressure to levels below 90 mmHg; our treatment of the SHR was far less effective, yet the disease was prevented and reversed by ACE inhibitor treatment and it was exacerbated by hydrochlorothiazide (that reduced arterial pressure to similar levels). And, fourth, it would seem (at least in the SHR) that antihypertensive therapy must have some degree of specificity in preventing and reversing ESRD. Thus, the ACE inhibitor and L-arginine did rapidly reverse the disease within three weeks pathologically and physiologically, whereas the thiazide enhanced the glomerular involvement. It is of particular interest that the ACE inhibitor achieves its effects by inhibiting the generation of angiotensin II systemically as well as locally within the kidney. On the other hand, the thiazide stimulates the renin-angiotensin system systemically and locally. Furthermore, there is an interaction of endothelially generated nitric oxide with angiotensin II and bradykinin (and these humoral substances are directly inhibited and generated by the ACE inhibitor, respectively). Thus, while these studies provide no information that directly pertains to patients with essential hypertension, the findings are appealing, important, and clearly relative to the widespread clinical problem.

Supporting Clinical Data

While there have been no independent studies or multicenter trials conducted in patients with essential hypertension that are relative to the above studies in the SHR or which can be extrapolated clinically, there have been some important clinical studies that are similar and germane. These studies have been conducted in normotensive as well as hypertensive patients with diabetes mellitus and renal parenchymal and vascular involvement from diabetes. These studies were conducted by treating some of the patients with an ACE inhibitor (e.g., captopril, ramipril) and others without that drug. The results of these studies clearly demonstrated that ACE inhibition therapy can reverse and retard the progression of diabetic renal disease in both normotensive and hypertensive patients.

There are a number of ongoing studies in patients with hypertension as well as with diabetes mellitus that have been designed to determine whether ACE inhibition, angiotensin II (type I) receptor antagonists, or calcium antagonists are able to reverse hypertensive renal disease and, hence, prevent the development of ESRD. These results are clearly anxiously anticipated.

Microalbuminuria

In recent years, it has been possible to assess more precisely microquantitative amounts of the daily urinary excretion of albumin. The risk of developing parenchymal renal involvement from essential hypertension by microalbuminuria determination has not yet been determined, although microalbuminuria has been related to ultimate morbidity and mortality of coronary heart disease (CHD). Nevertheless, the value of this determination is most important in assessing renal parenchymal involvement from primary renal diseases as well as for those patients with secondary renal involvement from such diseases as diabetes mellitus. Under the conditions of this method, normal albumin excretion is 30 to 300 mg/day (or 20 to 200 μg/min). At present, the method is relatively expensive (when one compares present costs for the conventional albumin excretion by "dipstick" or quantitative measurements with 24-hour urine collection), but advanced technology should soon simplify the technique and reduce cost. Indeed, such methodology is in clinical study and evaluation at this time.

Hyperuricemia

The phenomenon of hyperuricemia in patients with hypertension is extremely common, and it is not necessarily associated with gout or abnormal urate metabolism. A number of years ago we demonstrated that the height of serum uric acid concentration was directly related to the height of renal vascular resistance and the decrease in renal blood flow in patients with essential hypertension in patients of "borderline" and stage 1 and 2 severity. Moreover, the higher the patients' total peripheral resistance and the lower the cardiac output, the higher the serum uric acid concentration. These findings were analogous to an earlier clinical report which demonstrated that increased uric acid levels in response to norepinephrine or angiotensin II infusion into normotensive subjects were subsequently reversed upon discontinuing either pressor infusion. Our findings relating renal hemodynamic changes to the elevation of serum uric acid levels were subsequently confirmed in other controlled experimental studies in our laboratory. Thus, uric acid is a substance that is not only related to urate metabolism, but is also related to altered renal hemodynamics. Uric acid is delivered to the kidney as a function of renal blood flow, and it is filtered by the glomerulus and then absorbed and secreted by the tubule. In part, these fuctions are related to blood flow to the nephron.

Other studies in our clinical laboratory also indicated that in essential hypertensive patients without elevation of serum creatinine concentrations or without ECG evidence of LVH, uric acid predicts renal hemodynamic involvement in hypertension, but LVH predates these renal changes. Thus, those patients with echocardiographic evidence of LVH demonstrated no evidence of reduced renal blood flow or renal fraction of cardiac output (less than 17 percent of cardiac output) distributed to the kidney. However, if there was such evidence of reduced renal distribution of cardiac output, all of those patients had echocardiographic evidence of LVH. Moreover, when the uric acid concentration was elevated (greater than 6.5 and 8.5 mg/dL in women and men, respectively), the renal fraction of the cardiac output was significantly reduced and there was clear-cut echocardiographic evidence of LVH. Hence, it seems evident to me that hyperuricemia in untreated patients with essential hypertension represents an important index of renal involvement by nephrosclerosis. Moreover, the common clinical finding of hyperuricemia in untreated patients with essential hypertension or in patients with CHD is a risk factor that is an important surrogate of systemic and renal hemodynamic alterations (Figure 8.7).

An Integrated Concept

It is appropriate at this time to provide an integrated concept of the foregoing experimental and clinical findings related to our extant clinical knowledge concerning the pathophysiological mechanisms that may be related to the development of ESRD in patients with essential hypertension. Like other discussions in this monograph on hypertension, it would appear that there is a myriad of factors that seem to participate in the pathogenesis of ESRD in patients with essential hypertension. As with the other mosaic concepts (i.e., left ventricular hypertrophy, hyperuricemia, and essential hypertension per se), there are a number of clinical and pathophysiological factors that comprise a mosaic that relate as a kaleidoscope. Each of the factors are interdependent with the others in the pathogenesis of ESRD (Figure 8.8). Clearly, the elevated arterial pressure and the associated hemodynamic alterations that affect glomerular dynamics and capillary permeability are key determinants. These factors pertain to the increased glomerular hydrostatic pressure that results from afferent as well as efferent arteriolar constriction, even in the face of effective whole-kidney and single-nephron ischemia and reduced glomerular filtration rate. Also participating is the relationship of the disease with the aging process, racial and gender factors, and comorbid diseases, including atherosclerosis, diabetes mellitus, and hyperlipidemia. No doubt other factors, such as the renin-angiotensin system, humoral and growth factors, immune mechanisms, pharmacological agents, and local vascular mechanisms (including free radicals and the endothelial nitric oxide system), participate importantly. We already know, for example, that the endothelial generation of nitric oxide is markedly

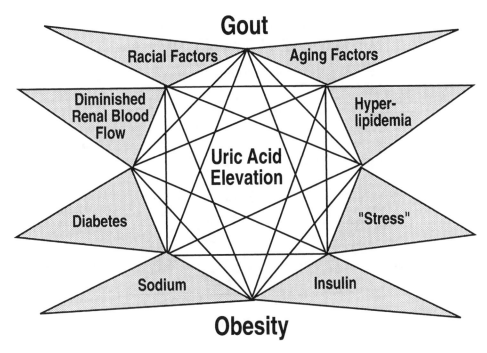

Figure 8.7. A mosaic of factors that seem to be related to hyperuricemia in patients with hypertension. (From Frohlich ED: Classic Papers Symposium History of Medicine Series: Surrogate indexes of target organ involvement in hypertension. *Am J Med Sci* 1996;312:225–228.

altered with aging, atherosclerosis, and hypertension. This was clearly demonstrated in the series of studies described above in the SHR. There is a close interrelationship between endothelially generated nitric oxide, bradykinin, and angiotensin II which obviously has its therapeutic counterparts. Hence, even though the amount of clinical data on renoprotection and treatment of nephrosclerosis in patients with essential hypertension is presently lacking, we are just beginning to find practical and beneficial clinical therapeutic effects in diabetic nephropathy. Hence, this discussion has been included.

SPECIFIC THERAPEUTIC RECOMMENDATIONS

Renoprotective Therapy

At the present time, there are no prospective clinical studies reported that suggest the value of specific antihypertensive therapy for patients with renal involvement and essential hypertension. As has been discussed, information is available that suggests that (1) strict blood pressure control may significantly slow the rate of impairment of renal function from patients with essential hypertension (e.g., MRFIT and HDFP studies) as well as from other target organs and (2) the ACE inhibitors have been shown to preserve renal function and reduce the degree of proteinuria in patients with insulin-dependent

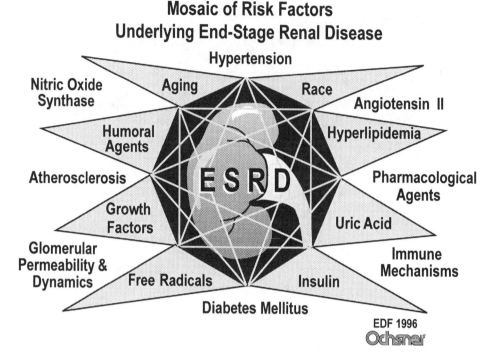

Figure 8.8.   Mosaic of risk factors that are involved in patients with hypertensions. (From Frohlich ED: 1996 Arthur C. Corcoran Lecture: Influence of nitric oxide and angiotensin II on renal involvement in hypertension. *Hypertension* 1997;29:188–193).

as well as non-insulin-dependent diabetes mellitus; but thus far, the available literature does not support the thesis that neither renal protection is provided nor is renal failure slowed by antihypertensive therapy. Perhaps this rather negative statement may be offset, in part, by the section above in which I have detailed our promising experimental experiences with various modes of antihypertensive therapy in our micropuncture studies.

Treatment of Hypertension in Patients with Renal Parenchymal Diseases

At this time, the major emphasis for antihypertensive therapy in essential hypertensive patients with parenchymal and functional involvement of the kidney is prompt recognition of the existence of hypertension and, then, the introduction of rigorous control of arterial pressure. Certainly, if the hypertensive patient is black or has hypertension associated with proteinuria and diabetic nephropathy, judicious use of ACE inhibitors associated with close monitoring of arterial pressure, renal function (serum creatinine and/or blood urea nitrogen concentrations), and serum potassium concentration is of extreme value. Because of the fluid retention associated with loss of renal function, addition of diuretics may be indicated, remembering that the lower doses are always preferable to higher doses. The thiazides are recommended until more severe compromise of renal function occurs; thereafter, the loop-acting agents (e.g., furosemide) are indicated. If, for any reason, the ACE inhibitors or the angiotensin II (type 1) receptor antagonists cannot be administered, then those calcium antagonists (e.g., diltiazem, verapamil, nitrendipine, felodipine) that appear to have beneficial actions on the kidney can be used alone or with the diuretics. Clearly when non-responding ESRD is apparent, long-term dialysis and renal transplantation must be considered.

Medical Treatment of Renovascular Hypertension

As suggested in the above discussion of renal arterial disease and hypertension, some hypertensive patients with renal arterial disease may be selected for medical treatment. This may be elected if (a) the physician wishes to follow a patient with renovascular hypertension for a time with medical therapy alone because the rate of progression of disease is not known, (b) the patient declines surgical or angioplasty therapy, or (c) the blood pressure is deemed well-controlled on existing antihypertensive therapy. As suggested in that earlier discussion, certain types of renal arterial lesions are known to progress very slowly and, hence, specific classes of antihypertensive drug therapy may be selected until such time that surgery or angioplasty is indicated. This may be dictated by the inability to provide adequate blood pressure control with antihypertensive drugs or when specific surgical complications of the renal arterial disease become manifest (e.g., dissection, further occlusion, hemorrhage). It is evident that the ACE inhibitors or angiotensin II (type 1) receptor antagonists would be first used for the patient with an angiotensin-dependent form of hypertension. This therapy could be augmented, if necessary, with the addition of a diuretic. However, if a patient has bilateral renal arterial disease or unilateral renal arterial disease in a solitary kidney, the ACE inhibitors are contraindicated. In this latter situation, in my experience, the use of a calcium antagonist (e.g., diltiazem or verapamil) is clearly indicated and of great value.

Surgical Treatment

When the managing physician decides that surgical repair of the renal arterial lesion is indicated, this may be approached either by angioplasty or by surgical correction of the renal arterial lesion depending upon the specific circumstances of that renal arterial lesion. In selecting either therapy, one must bear in mind the possibility of the potential development of arterial disease in the same or in the contralateral kidney. Hence, the approach to such treatment should be entertained very carefully and discussed in detail with available consultants. The options range from the possible need for nephrectomy or autonephrectomy, renal arterial bypass surgery, arterial grafting, or endarterectomy to removal of the arterial segment with the lesion and then end-to end anastomosis of the artery. Space does not permit more detailed discussion of these surgical options; a detailed text is referred to at the end of this chapter. However, an additional word is indicated with respect to preoperative preparations. In general, I prefer that prior to surgery an isotopic renogram is obtained in order to obtain baseline information should postoperative problems occur (e.g., development of severe hypertension, possibility of postoperative occlusion of the renal artery) that requires a more immediate postoperative renogram for comparison. On the day of surgical procedure, the patient could be given the usual antihypertensive medication with a sip of water; and, then, if the patient requires antihypertensive drug therapy postoperatively, it can be maintained orally or parenterally (using the same agent or class of agents). Finally, it is important to remember that if renal arterial surgery is performed, that arterial pressure should be well controlled postoperatively in order to prevent strain at the arterial suture lines and hemorrhage.

ANNOTATED BIBLIOGRAPHY

References that provide excellent resources to understand the natural history of the various renal arterial diseases

1. McCormick LJ, Poutasse EF, Meaney TF, Noto TJ, Dustan HP: A pathologic–arteriographic correlation of renal arterial disease. *Am Heart J* 1966;72:188–198.
2. Schreiber MJ, Pohl MA, Novick AC: The natural history of atherosclerotic and fibrous renal artery disease. *Urol Clin North Am* 1984;11:383–392.
3. Tollefson DFJ, Ernst CB: Natural history of atherosclerotic renal artery stenosis associated with aortic disease. *J Vasc Surg* 1991;14:327–331.
   Selected references of diagnostic studies to evaluate presence of renal arterial disease.
4. Mann SJ, Pickering TG: Detection of renovascular hypertension. State of the art: 1992. *Ann Intern Med* 1992;117:845–853.
5. Andersen GH, Blakeman N, Streeten DHP: Prediction of renovascular hypertension. Comparison of clinical diagnostic indices. *Am J Hypertens* 1988; 1:301–304.
6. Blaufox MD, Middleton ML, Bonogiovanni J, Davis BR: Cost efficacy of the diagnosis and therapy of renovascular hypertension. *J Nucl Med* 1996; 37:171–177.
7. Vidt DG: The diagnosis of renovascular hypertension: a clinician's viewpoint. *Am J Hypertens* 1991;4(suppl):663–668.
8. Dondi M: Captopril renal scintigraphy with ^{99m}Tcmercaptoacetyltriglycine (^{99m}Tc-MAG$_3$) for detecting renal artery stenosis. *Am J Hypertens* 1991;4(suppl): 737–740.
9. Burns PN. The physical principles of Doppler and spectral analysis. *J Clin Ultrasound* 1987;15:567–590.
10. Hansen KJ, Tribble RW, Reavis SW, et al: Duplex ultrasound scanning in the diagnosis of renal artery stenosis: a prospective evaluation. *J Vasc Surg* 1988; 7:363–369.
11. Kim D, Edelman RR, Kent KC, Porter DH, Skillman JJ: Abdominal aorta and renal artery stenosis: Evaluation with MR angiography. *Radiology* 1990;174: 727–731.
12. Sondergaard L, Stohlberg F, Thomsen C, Stensgaard A, Lindvig K, Henriksen O. Accuracy and precision of MR velocity mapping in measurement of stenotic cross-sectional area, flow rate, and pressure gradient. *J Magn Reson Imaging* 1993;3:433–437.
13. Rubin GD, Walker PJ, Dake MD, et al. Three-dimensional spiral computed tomographic angiography: an alternative imaging modality for the abdominal aortic and its branches. *J Vasc Surg* 1993;18:656–665.
14. Pohl MA: Renovascular hypertension: An internist's point of view. In: *Hypertension* (Punzi H, Flamembaum W, eds). Futura Publishing Co, New York, 1989, p. 367.
    References concerned with treatment of renal arterial disease
15. Tegtmeyer CJ, Hartwell GD, Selby JB, Robertson R Jr, Kron IL, Tribble CG: Results and complications of angioplasty in aortoiliac disease. *Circulation* 1991;83(Suppl I):53–60.

16. Puijaert CBAJ, Boomsma JHB, Ruijs JHJ, et al: Transluminal renal artery dilatation in hypertension: Technique, results, and complications in 60 cases. *Urol Radiol* 1981;2:201–210.
17. Novick AC: Management of renovascular disease: a surgical perspective. *Circulation* 1991;83(Suppl I):167–171.
18. Sos TA: Angioplasty for the treatment of azotemia and renovascular hypertension in atherosclerotic renal artery disease. *Circulation* 1991;83(Suppl I):162–166. General references concerned with end stage renal disease
19. Spitalewitz S, Weber MA, Reiser IW: Medical and non-medical approaches to renovascular hypertension. *Cardiologia* 1997;42:237–243.
20. Dustan HP: Renal arterial disease and hypertension. In: *Essential Hypertension,* (Frohlich ED, editor) *Medical Clin N America* 1997;81:1199–1212. General references concerned with end-stage renal disease
21. National High Blood Pressure Education Program Working Group: 1995 Update of the Working Group Reports on Chronic Renal Failure and Renovascular Hypertension. *Arch Intern Med* 1996;156:1938–1947.
22. Blyth WB, Maddux FW: Hypertension as a causative diagnosis of patients entering end-stage renal disease programs in the United States from 1980 to 1986. *Am J Kidney Dis* 1991;18:33–37.
23. U.S. Renal Data Systems: 1995 Annual Data Report. National Institutes of Health, National Institute of Diabetes, Digestive and Kidney Diseases. III. Incidence and causes of treated ESRD. *Am J Kidney Dis* 1995;26:S39–S50.
24. Frohlich ED: 1996 Arthur C. Corcoran Lecture: Influence of nitric oxide and angiotensin II on renal involvement in hypertension. *Hypertension* (1997;29: 188–193.
25. Rostand SG: US minority groups and end-stage renal disease: A disproportionate share. *Am J Kidney Dis* 1992;19:411–413.
26. Perry HM, Miller JP, Fornoff JR, et al: Early predictors of 15-year end-stage renal disease in hypertensive patients. *Hypertension* 1995;25:587–594.
27. Perneger TV, Whelton PK, Klag MJ: Race and end-stage renal disease: Socioeconomic status and access to health care as mediating factors. *Arch Intern Med* 1995;155:1201–1208.
28. Epstein M, Sower JR: Diabetes mellitus and hypertension. *Hypertension* 1992;19:403–418.
29. Hollenberg NK, Borucki LJ, Adams DF: The renal vasculature in early essential hypertension: Evidence for a pathogenic role. *Medicine* 1978;57:167–178.
30. Brenner BM, Meyer TW, Hostetter TH: Dietary protein intake and the progressive nature of kidney disease: The tale of hemodynamically mediated glomerular disease in the pathogenesis of progressive glomerular sclerosis in aging, renal ablation, and intrinsic renal disease. *N Engl J Med* 1982;307:652–659.
31. Hostetter TH, Olson JL, Rennke HG, Venkatachalam MA, Brenner BM: Hyperfiltration in remnant nephros: A potentially adverse response to renal ablation. *Am J Physiol* 1981;241:F85–F93.
32. Frohlich ED, Messerli FH, Oigman W, Ventura HO, Sundgaard-Riise K: Greater renal vascular involvement in the black patient with essential hypertension. *Miner Electrolyte Metab* 1984;10:173–177.
33. Raij L, Baylis C: Glomerular actions of nitric oxide. *Kidney Int* 1995;48:20–32. Effect of treatment on hypertensive end-stage renal disease

34. National High Blood Pressure Education Program Working Group: National High Blood Pressure Education Program working group report on hypertension and diabetes. *Hypertension* 1994;23:145–158.

35. Berg R, Buckalew V, Pearce G, Poruch J, Rauch S, Schulman G, for the MDRD Study Group: Differences between hypertensive and normotensive patients in the Modification of Diet in Renal Disease Study (MDRD) cohort. Presented at the Twelfth International Congress of Nephrology, June 13–18, 1993, Jerusalem, Israel. Abstract, p. 594.

36. Lewis EJ, Hunsicker LG, Bain RP, Rhode RD, for the Collaborative Study Group. The effect of angiotensin-converting-enzyme inhibition on diabetic nephropathy. *N Engl J Med* 1993;329:1456–1462.

37. Zucchelli P, Zuccala A, Borghi M, et al: Long-term comparison between captopril and nifedipine in the progression of renal insufficiency. *Kidney Int* 1992;42:452–458.

38. Bauer JH, Reams GP, Lal SM: Renal protective effect of strict blood pressure control with enalapril therapy. *Arch Intern Med* 1987;147:1397–1400.

39. Pettinger WA, Lee HC, Reisch J, Mitchell HC. Long-term improvement in renal function after short-term strict blood pressure control in hypertensive nephrosclerosis. *Hypertension* 1989;13:766–772.

40. Bakris GL, Barnhill BW, Sadler R. Treatment of arterial hypertension in diabetic humans: importance of therapeutic selection. *Kidney Int* 1992;41:912–919.

41. Shulman NB, Ford CE, Hall D, Blaufox MD, Simon D, Langford HG, et al: Prognostic value of serum creatinine and effect of treatment of hypertension on renal function: Results from the Hypertension Detection and Follow-up Program. *Hypertenison* 1989;13(Suppl I):180–193.

42. Pettinger WA, Lee HC, Reisch J, Mitchell HC: Long-term improvement in renal function after short-term strict blood pressure control in hypertenisve nephrosclerosis. *Hypertension* 1989;13:766–772.

43. Kasiske BL, Kalil RSN, Ma JZ, Liao M, Keane WM: Effects of antihypertensive therapy on the kidney in patients with diabetes: A meta-regression analysis. *Ann Intern Med* 1993;118:129–138.

44. Stanton JR, Freis ED: Serum uric acid concentration in essential hypertenison. *Proc Soc Exp Biol Med* 1947;66:193–194.
    Role of serum uric acid concentration in hypertension is discussed in the following five references.

45. Messerli FH, Frohlich ED, Dreslinski GR, Suarez DH, Aristimuño GG: Serum uric acid in essential hypertension: An indicator of renal vascular involvement. *Ann Intern Med* 1980;93:817–821.

46. Kobrin I, Frohlich, ED, Ventura, HO, Messerli FH: Renal involvement follows cardiac enlargement in essential hypertension. *Arch Intern Med* 1986;146:272–276.

47. Nunez BD, Frohlich ED, Garavaglia GE, Schmieder RE, Nunez MM: Serum uric acid in renovascular hypertension: Reduction following surgical correction. *Am J Med Sci* 1987;294:419–422.

48. Sesoko S, Pegram BL, Willis GW, Frohlich ED: DOCA-salt induced malignant hypertension in spontaneously hypertensive rats. *J Hypertens* 1984;2:49–54.

Chapter 9

Approaches to the Treatment of Patients with Stroke and Hypertensive Emergencies

If there is one group of vascular complications of hypertension that has been dramatically reduced as a result of antihypertensive therapy, it is that due to stroke and hypertensive emergencies. Over the past 25 years, there has been a dramatic reduction in deaths from stroke (upwards of 70 percent). Moreover, as indicated earlier in this text, hospital admissions for the variety of problems heretofore termed "hypertensive emergencies" has also decreased to what may be considered clinical rarities. Thus, whereas these and some of the other major and devastating illnesses related to hypertension had accounted for the majority of hospital admissions two or three decades ago, they are much less commonly encountered today. This is not to suggest by any stretch of the imagination that one does not encounter these problems today. We certainly do, but the number and variety of diagnostic "tools" and therapeutic "weapons" have so increased that the problem is far less frustrating and dismal than what we have experienced in the past.

STROKE

The one major clear-cut benefit of the early recognition and vigorous treatment of hypertension has been the ability to effect a striking reduction of stroke, whether hemorrhagic, thrombotic, embolic, or rupture of the very small cerebral Charcot–Beuchard aneurysms. Nevertheless, one must also bear in mind the reality that strokes are also common in the majority of our population (over 75 percent) who do not have systemic arterial hypertension. Notwithstanding this moderating thought are three important considerations: (1) hypertension is responsible for most of the strokes in the United States and the decline in stroke deaths; (2) black patients are particularly predisposed to strokes; and (3) the decline of death rates and incidence rates of stroke in the United States appear to be leveling off (and, perhaps, even starting to increase). Furthermore, still remaining as an exceedingly common complication in normotensive and hypertensive individuals are the so-called "small strokes." These abnormalities may also result from embolic disease from atherosclerotic plaques of the great vessels, rupture of smallCharcot–Beuchard aneurysms, or small thrombi in the smaller arteries of the cerebral circulation. These facets of the broader problem of stroke in hypertension will be discussed briefly.

General

First, although this thought should be obvious, not every patient with hypertension and stroke constitutes a hypertensive emergency. Thus, although the acute development of a stroke resulting from the thrombosis of an artery in the cerebral circulation may result in sudden loss of consciousness, total or partial paralysis, or total or partial loss of sensory modalities, it does not constitute a hypertensive emergency, per se. Clearly, it may be a true medical emergency but may not necessarily be one of a hypertensive emergency that requires immediate and rapid blood pressure reduction. On the other hand, a sudden subarachnoid hemorrhage resulting from a ruptured cerebral aneurysm (in the circle of Willis), an intracerebral hemorrhage, or a cerebral embolus in a hypertensive patient may be a real hypertensive emergency that should be approached more dramatically. In any event, as with many of the issues relating to hypertension and its complications, there are a number of underlying factors that contribute to the overall risk of the patient with hypertension in developing a stroke (Figure 9.1).

Evaluation of the Patient

In an earlier chapter (Chapter 2) we have dealt in some detail with the clinical evaluation of the hypertensive patient. Only a few points demand further elaboration with

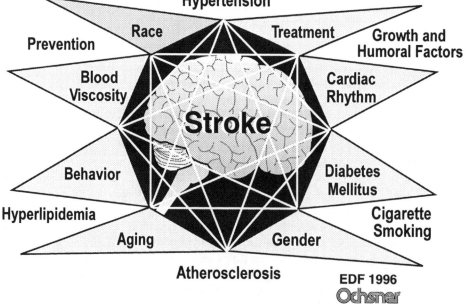

Figure 9.1. The multifactorial nature of the risk factors underlying stroke.

regard to stroke. With respect to issues relating to the patient's history, it is vitally important to know whether there is a family history of cerebral hemorrhage. A family history of aneurysmal disease is significant, since a history of hepatic or renal cystic disease and coexisting polycythemia constitutes a genetically transmitted syndrome. Also of critical importance is the drug history of the patient. Sudden discontinuance of antihypertensive therapy is vitally important, particularly in those patients who had been taking clonidine, methyldopa, or beta-adrenergic receptor blocking drugs. While not as common today, arterial pressure rebounds precipitously following abrupt cessation of these drugs and may thereby be responsible for a stroke. Furthermore, in those patients receiving monoamine oxidase inhibitors (not only for hypertension but also isoniazid for tuberculosis as well as certain agents for psychiatric illness), ingestion of certain foodstuffs containing tyramine (e.g., chianti wine, certain cheeses, and marinated foods) may be responsible for a sudden release of norepinephrine from nerve endings and elsewhere. The released norepinephrine does not became metabolized rapidly, and the sudden rise in arterial pressure may be associated with stroke. And, of course, there is the unfortunately common use of "street drugs" (e.g., cocaine, heroin, morphine) which may also produce a pressor crisis and stroke.

A complete physical examination is clearly essential. This includes the careful inspection of the optic fundi for evidence of embolic disease, papilledema, hemorrhages, and exudates. Cardiac examination must be performed with care, and notation should be made as to the rhythm since atrial fibrillation or runs of ectopic beats should suggest the very real possibility of embolic disease. Moreover, the remainder of the examination should also include careful exploration for other evidence of embolic phenomena. Clearly, the neurological examination must be performed in detail. It is essential that the physician note (on the patient's record) carefully the state of sensorium of the patient on admission and frequently thereafter, so that therapeutic management of the patient is made less complex. Thus, some antihypertensive (or other prescribed) therapy may obtund the sensorium, thereby vastly complicating the overall management of the patient and the disease.

In this day and age, the admitting physician usually can arrange for an immediate CAT scan of the brain once the severely elevated pressure is controlled. This study not infrequently may resolve the issue of thrombosis versus hemorrhage. However, there still may be the need for performance of a lumbar puncture. If a lumbar puncture is performed, it is not necessary to obtain a large amount of fluid for special studies; but a small amount may be extremely valuable for resolving the issue of thrombosis versus hemorrhage. Thus, if the spinal tap was traumatic, the fluid which was immediately "spun down" in a nearby centrifuge should have a clear supernatant. However, if the patient sustained a subarachnoid hemorrhage, the spinal fluid that was centrifuged would appear xanthochromic as a result of prior red blood cell hemolysis. Furthermore, as soon as the possibility of subarachnoid hemorrhage is entertained, it is advisable to notify the appropriate neurosurgical consultant in order to minimize the valuable time necessary for this evaluation and disposition of the problem.

The next major point for clinical resolution is whether the patient has had preexisting hypertension with the subsequent complication of stroke from cerebral thrombosis or whether that patient with hypertension requires more vigorous and careful control of arterial pressure. This is exceedingly important since inherent in this decision is the approach to further blood pressure management: immediate careful reduction of arterial pressure elevation, the type of antihypertensive therapy to be prescribed, whether the patient requires a continuous intravenous infusion of anti-hypertensive medication with monitoring of arterial pressure, and whether the patient should be admitted to a specific type of acute care unit.

Treatment

Once the foregoing clinical decisions are made, then the critical question remains: Just what antihypertensive agent should be selected from the vast number of options that are presently available (Table 9.1). If the physician feels that the pressure in the stroke patient is severely elevated and requires control, several issues must be resolved. First, if the patient is known to have had hypertension in the past and the blood pressure has been under good control up until the occurrence of the stroke or if the blood pressure is only slightly elevated at the time of hospital admission with stroke, the previously prescribed antihypertensive medications should be continued (providing, of course, the patient is able to take medications by mouth).

On the other hand, if the blood pressure is clearly out of control or if the patient cannot take medications by mouth, there are two possibilities: Either the patient had not taken the prescribed medications or the blood pressure is no longer being adequately controlled with the medications prescribed previously. If the former is the case, then the earlier prescribed medications should be reinstituted and the blood pressures should be carefully monitored. If, on the other hand, arterial pressure had not been controlled, then there are two subsequent options depending on whether the patient is able to take medications by mouth or by intravenous route. In the former instance, medications should be instituted and the blood pressure should be controlled, but not with the immediate goal of precipitous pressure reduction. If, however, the patient requires par-

TABLE 9.1. Antihypertensive Agents for Acute Hypertensive Emergencies[a]

Diuretics:	Chlorothiazide (iv, po)
	Furosemide (iv, po)
Direct vascular	Diazoxide (iv)
smooth muscle	Sodium nitroprusside (iv)
relaxants:	Hydralazine (iv, im, po)
Alpha Adrenergic	Nitroglycerine (iv)
Receptor Blockers	Dibenzylene (iv)
	Phenoxybenzamine (po)
Adrenolytic Agents	Methyldopa (iv, po)
	Reserpine (im, sub-Q, po)
	Trimethaphan camsylate (iv)
	Cryptenamine (iv)
Beta Adrenergic	Propranolol (iv, po)
Receptor Blockers:	Esmolol (iv)
Alpha/Beta Adrenergic	Labetalol (iv, po)
Receptor Blockers:	
ACE inhibitors:	Lisinopril (iv, po)
Calcium antagonists:	Diltiazem (iv, po)
	Verapamil (iv, po)
	Nicardipine (iv, po)
Dopamine Agonist	Fenoldapam (iv)

[a]Nifedipine capsules *not* included nor indicated. iv, intravenously; im, intramuscularly; po, orally.

enterally administered antihypertensive medications, this should be done with extreme care and slowly and with close monitoring of arterial pressure (Table 9.2).

Recently, neurologists have completed double-blinded, placebo-controlled studies that indicate immediate treatment with the intravenous thrombolytic agent TPA will reduce the residual from stroke. At this time, at least to the thinking of this author, its use in the hypertensive patient with stroke is still unresolved, and there is still clear cut risk of cerebral bleeding in these patients. Nevertheless, chronic anti-thrombotic therapy with aspirin (or its equivalents) or dipyridimole is a very wise intervention to prevent subsequent events.

Rapid, but well-controlled, blood pressure can be achieved with intravenous sodium nitroprusside or trimethaphan camsylate; less control might be achieved with intravenous labetalol or diltiazem. More prolonged arterial pressure control with nitroprusside may be complicated by intravolume expansion and subsequent loss of that pressure control. However, reinstitution of that blood pressure control can be restored with the intravenous administration of a diuretic (e.g., furosemide, chlorothiazide), but there should also be careful monitoring of serum potassium concentration. Prolonged blood pressure control with nitroprusside may be complicated by symptoms of thiocyanate toxicity which can be confirmed by measurement of thiocyanate levels. On the other hand, trimethapham may be complicated by intestinal ileus. It is of vital importance to reiterate that use of more prolonged intravenous antihypertensive drugs is offset by the difficulty in maintaining moment-to-moment control of blood pressure. (For further discussion the reader is referred to chapters 4 and 5.)

In any patient who had been normotensive or had hypertensive disease under good blood pressure control, but then had a sudden elevation of arterial pressure with or without the associated hypertensive complication (such as stroke), it is important to consider the possibility of secondary causes of hypertension (e.g., possible lack of adherence to an antihypertensive treatment program, development of an occlusive renal arterial lesion). This investigation should be pursued as soon as it is clinically feasible. It goes without saying that renal arteriography would only be pursued as soon as the patient has stabilized in the hospital and the blood pressure is controlled.

Consultations

In this respect, it is of utmost importance (when indicated) to secure expert consultative advice concerning blood pressure control in the areas of radiology, neurosurgery,

---

Table 9.2. Rapid (and Controlled) Blood Pressure Reduction

- Contolled intravenous infusion
  - Sodium nitroprusside
  - Labetalol hydrochloride
  - Trimethaphane camsylate
  - Lisinopril
  - Propranolol hydrochloride or esmolol (primarily for catecholamine-induced arrhythmias)
  - Fenoldopam mesylate
- Slow addition of oral agents as the clinical situation
- If only by the intravenous port, beware of the development of "pseudotolerance" and add diuretic as needed

as well as in the physical medicine, and rehabilitation. Indeed, it follows that the earlier this latter consultative advice is obtained, the sooner appropriate rehabilitation can be initiated. It goes without saying that if the stroke was produced by a suspected ruptured cerebral artery aneurysm, four vessel arteriographic studies should be obtained to supplement prior CAT scanning or magnetic resonance imaging information. However, even before arteriographic procedures are pursued, it is also wise to contact the most experienced neurosurgical consultant available about repair of a bleeding cerebral arterial aneurysm and the prevention of subsequent aneurysmal ruptures. On the other hand, if the cerebral bleeding was produced by an intracerebral bleeding episode, then neurological, neurosurgical, and physical medical consultative advice should also be obtained with the aim of salvaging the patient with minimal physical disability and hospitalization.

Atrial Fibrillation

Finally, if stroke occurs in a patient with atrial fibrillation, the managing physician should immediately consider the possibility that the stroke was caused by an embolism from the heart. In this case, the complete differential diagnosis of the cardiac or other diseases must be considered. This should include possibilities of thyrotoxicosis, valvular heart disease, or any of the other comorbid conditions that may be associated with atrial fibrillation. In this case, one of the earlier therapeutic decisions which must be faced is the conversion of the atrial fibrillation to sinus rhythm and whether anticoagulants should be administered. This is an extremely difficult decision in the patient with hypertension, particularly if the blood pressure has not been under good control. Thus, in the patient with hypertension, especially if the pressure is not in optimal control, there is a greater chance for cerebral hemorrhage; this possibility must be considered. Personally, I am reluctant to prescribe anticoagulant therapy in the patient with hypertension, particularly if the pressure had not been in optimal control. This also includes the newer approaches and means for administering thrombolytic therapy to the patient with stroke. In its place I would consider administering aspirin or dipyridamole. In any event, conversion of the rhythm is extremely important; and, once this is done, in addition to antiarrhythmic therapy, daily aspirin and/or dipyridamole should be considered—particularly when anticoagulants are not employed.

ACUTE HYPERTENSIVE ENCEPHALOPATHY

This hypertensive emergency is much less frequently encountered these days, but it still occurs. It is manifested by a severely elevated arterial pressure that is associated with progressively more severe neurological signs and symptoms and rapid deterioration of the neurological disease from headache, nausea, vomiting, and sensory or motor deficits, leading to drowsiness and, then, to coma. The neurological findings are produced by intense arteriolar constriction in the brain which may be manifested by threadlike or even absent retinal arterioles on funduscopic examination. Effective treatment is by rapid (i.e., instantaneous) reduction of arterial pressure. This can be achieved by the intravenous injection of diazoxide, provided that there is no evidence of angina pectoris, cardiac failure, myocardial dissection, or aortic dissection. As indicated elsewhere in this text, in these foregoing situations, rapid reduction of arterial pressure with diazoxide or hydralazive will precipitate a reflexive stimulation of the heart and cardiovascular system so that those underlying cardiac and aortic conditions can be exacerbated, a fatal outcome may even result. Following this same line of reasoning, in no circumstance should this condition be treated with the capsular, rapidly acting formulation of the calcium antagonist nifedipine. That latter agent works no more rapidly than the other more appropriate agents; if rapid reduction of pressure is deemed necessary, this should be conducted as indicated above with intravenous nitroprusside or trimethaphan camsylate. The patient should be followed carefully in the intensive care setting where a more appropriate long-term agent can be selected, introduced, and used thereafter. It is of particular note that in the patient with acute hypertensive encephalopathy, associated with the rapid (i.e., immediate) reduction of arterial pressure, there is a rapid (an immediate) clearing of the neurological signs and symptoms with awakening of the patient from coma. As indicated above, as soon as arterial pressure is controlled and the patient can take oral medications, they should be prescribed and the patient should be returned to a regular hospital room.

ACCELERATED AND MALIGNANT HYPERTENSION

Although this severe and rapidly progressing form of hypertension is far less commonly encountered today than 20 years ago, it is still encountered and demands an enlightened approach to its management. The disease may be defined as a true hypertensive emergency that requires its prompt (i.e., within hours or one to two days) reduction and control of pressure. The disease is manifested by a high arterial pressure, but it should not be defined by a specific elevation of diastolic or systolic pressure. In the years prior to effective antihypertensive therapy, 97 percent of patients with malignant hypertension died within a few months. Now, the long-term picture is considerably improved, particularly in patients without severe renal and cardiac functional impairment.

Pathophysiology

The elevated arterial pressure in accelerated and malignant hypertension is produced by severe arteriolar constriction that produces its secondary effects (at least, in part) by intense renal arteriolar constriction and parenchymal ischemia. This initiates an increase in the release of renin by the juxtaglomerular cells which results in increased generation of angiotensin II and a secondary increase in aldosterone secretion from the adrenal cortex. The result is hyperreninemic secondary aldosteronism that is manifested by hypokalemic alkalosis (as described in Chapter 1). Pathologically, there is round cell infiltration of the renal arteriolar wall, deposition of complement in the renal parenchyma, marked proteinuria, elevated serum gammaglobulin concentration, and microangiopathic hemolytic anemia. Not infrequently, the problem may be associated with renal functional impairment (of varying degrees of severity), left ventricular hypertrophy, and even cardiac failure. The major point of differentiating the patient with accelerated hypertension from one with malignant hypertension is the presence of papilledema of the optic fundi and exudative retinopathy in patients with malignant hypertension. Patients with accelerated hypertension do not yet have papilledema, although there is evidence of exudative retinopathy (hemorrhages and exudates).

A question still exists as to the possible initiating events of malignant hypertension. Classically, clinicians have explored very vigorously the possibility of renovascular hypertension; this, no doubt, must be excluded—particularly if there is no evidence of renal functional impairment. Of course, if there is renal functional impairment, the disease would have to be based upon bilateral occlusive renal arterial disease. More frequently, however, there is no apparent secondary course for the hypertension although recent introduction of ACE inhibition therapy should always be considered and, if this is so, it should be immediately discontinued. (Parenthetically, I have often wondered whether there may be an autoimmune basis for this disease when one considers the features that are shared by malignant hypertension.)

In my opinion, there is less necessity for the patient to be admitted into an intensive care unit if there are no features of the problem that require more intensive supervision of the patients care than the close and frequent monitoring of blood pressure and other vital signs (including measurement of daily weights in order to detect fluid retention) and administration of the selected antihypertensive medications. If this be the case, the patient can be followed closely and carefully in a room adjacent to the nurses' station. In selecting an effective antihypertensive therapeutic program, the clinician must be aware of the problem of severe secondary hyperaldosteronism with its attendant hypokalemic alkalosis and hypomagnesemia and their complications. This means that careful monitoring of the patient's cardiac rhythm is essential.

Once bilateral renal arterial disease is excluded (and this can be done by isotopic renal flows and scans as well as by selective arteriography, doppler renal flows, etc.), administration of an ACE inhibitor is sound therapy. However, blood pressure should be followed very carefully for several hours after the first dose and before the dose is increased. A diuretic most likely will be essential, but the physician should be aware that the diuretic can exacerbate the hypokalemia and increase the chances of severe cardiac arrhythmias. To obviate this, administration of spironolactone is a wise choice; but this agent also may be associated with problems. On one hand, this is related to the problem of future hyperkalemia once the potassium-retaining agent is administered, particularly if the patient is also taking an ACE inhibitor. Hence, the serum potassium concentration must be followed carefully and, perhaps, along with the measurement of serum magnesium concentration. It may be wise to administer the ACE inhibitor initially in its intravenous formulation (e.g., lisinopril), and should this be pursued, then it would be wiser to have the patient followed (at least initially) in an intensive care setting where the infusion rate of the prescribed drug can be carefully monitored along with the level of arterial pressure (perhaps by intra-arterial measurement and monitoring). Once pressure is well controlled, the medication can be switched to the oral formulation of an ACE inhibitor.

If, however, an ACE inhibitor or an angiotensin II (type 1) receptor antagonist cannot be administered, then the administration of a calcium antagonist (e.g., diltiazem or verapamil) can be administered. Certainly, this would be the likely consideration if the patient is known to have bilateral renal arterial disease or unilateral renal arterial stenosis in a solitary kidney.

ACUTE PRESSOR CRISES

There are a number of hypertensive emergencies that will be described herein under the unifying term of "pressor crises." Each is a discrete clinical problem, but they all have a unifying theme that is related to an underlying mechanism(s). This mechanism is concerned with excessive participation of adrenergically mediate pressor phenomena (Table 9.3).

"Street Drugs"

With respect to the pressor crisis associated with the ingestion of so-called "street drugs," we refer to an increased arterial pressure typified by cocaine abuse. As we know from classical pharmacological studies, cocaine inhibits norepinephrine reuptake by the adrenergic nerve ending. As a result, arterial pressure rises and the heart suffers from excessive adrenergic stimulation. Treatment of the crisis is multifold: (1) cessation of the cocaine; (2) control of arterial pressure by parenteral (e.g., phenoxybenzamine) or oral (e.g., dibenzyline, doxazosine, prazosin, terazosine) alpha-adrenergic receptor inhibitors; (3) prevention or treatment of beta-adrenergically mediated cardiac arrhythmias (e.g., propranolol); and, of course,(4) long-term treatment of this horrible addiction. With today's practice of medicine the latter is by far the most difficult clinical (and social) problem.

Sudden Withdrawal of Adrenolytic Agents

A second adrenergically mediated pressor crisis results from the sudden discontinuance of one of the relatively short-acting centrally active alpha-receptor agonists (e.g., clonidine, methyldopa). Treatment follows a similar approach to that suggested above: discontinuance or immediate resumption of the adrenergic inhibitor and immediate control of the abrupt rise of pressure and associated cardiac arrhythmias with parenteral alpha- and beta-adrenergic receptor blockers, respectively.

MAO Inhibitors

In the case of the pressor crisis that is associated with monoamine oxidase (MAO) inhibitors, these agents inhibit the norepinephrine degradation after its release from the nerve ending. Thus, when the patient ingests certain foods that contain tyramine (e.g., Chianti wine, certain cheeses), norepinephrine is released from the nerve endings and

Table 9.3. Pressor Crises

Crisis	Rx
"Street drugs" (e.g., cocaine)	Cessation and alpha-blockers Beta and/or alpha-beta–blockers
Antihypertensive drug withdrawal (e.g., clonidine, methyldopa)	Reinstitution of Rx (?) and rapid control of pressure New treatment program Alpha or alpha-beta–blockers
MAO inhibitor therapy with ingestion of tyramine-containing foods	Alpha or alpha-beta–blockers
Guanethidine or guanadrel antihypertensive therapy associated with imipramine or desipramine antidepressants	Discontinue guanethidine or guanadrel
Pheochromocytoma	Alpha or alpha-beta–blockers

arterial pressure increases markedly without the necessary rapid metabolism of the released catecholamine. The treatment of the pressor crisis is also similar to the means described above.

Guanethidine and Imipramine

Still another pressor crisis relates to the patient who has been taking a postganglionic neuronal blocking agent such as guanethidine or guanadril. These agents deplete the nerve ending of norepinephrine which is then replaced by one of these antihypertensive agents. Then, if the patient also suffers from depression and is treated with either imipramine or desimipramine, the antidepressant prevents neuronal uptake of the antihypertensive agents and arterial pressure also rises abruptly. The treatment, again, is very similar to that described above.

Pheochromocytoma

Finally, another important pressor crisis involving similar adrenergic mechanisms relate to the sudden discharge of catecholamines from pheochromocytoma tumor. As a result, arterial pressure rises from the alpha-adrenergic stimulation of receptors on the vessel wall, and cardiac disrhythmias result from beta-adrenergic stimulation of the cardiac myocytes. Arterial pressure may remain continuously elevated, or pressor crises may be precipitated by sudden falls of arterial pressure, physical stimulation of the tumor that releases catecholamines from the tumor, or administration of a hyperostotic solution (e.g., radiographic contrast material). The treatment of the pressure rise is also with injectable alpha- and beta-adrenergic receptor inhibitors. Surgical removal of the tumor is not to be pursued on an emergent basis. Rather, prior treatment with a long-acting alpha-adrenergic receptor inhibition drug will provide (a) control of pressure reexpansion of the associated intravascular volume and (b) minimization of intraoperative pressor crises.

ACUTE PULMONARY EDEMA AND CARDIAC FAILURE

Hypertension associated with acute pulmonary edema and congestive heart failure should be treated with parenterally administered drugs. Immediate use of thigh "cuffs," intravenous diuretics, and digoxin may be indicated (depending upon the severity of the acute problem). An ACE inhibitor will reduce left ventricular preloads and afterloads. If the ACE inhibitor is not effective, it is worthwhile to initiate therapy with the smooth muscle relaxant sodium nitroprusside which also reduces left ventricular preload and afterload. It is also important to remember that when the diuretic is administered to this patient with secondary hyperaldosteronism (resulting from cardiac failure), it may be associated with exacerbation of the cardiac arrhythmias related to hypokalemia and/or hypomagnesemia.

AORTIC COARCTATION AND POSTVASCULAR SURGERY

It is also essential to control an elevated arterial pressure in patients following coronary arterial bypass surgery, repair of aortic aneurysm, aortic coarctation, or any other cardiovascular surgery. This is best achieved by administration of sodium nitroprusside in the surgical intensive postoperative care setting since this means for arterial pressure reduction is not associated with reflex stimulation of the heart and provides continuous monitoring of the pressure.

Similarly, in patients with dissecting aortic aneurysm, it is necessary to reduce arterial pressure rapidly without reflexively stimulating the heart and thereby exacerbate the aortic dissection process. As pressure declines, the chest or back pain rapidly abates. At this point, it is necessary to establish the dissection arteriographically or by noninvasive Doppler sonographic techniques while obtaining appropriate cardiovascular surgical consultation. A similar concept may be advanced for the patient with a severely elevated arterial pressure following repair of aortic coarctation or acute myocardial infarction. Arterial pressure must be well controlled without unduly reducing the pressure to levels so that diastolic perfusion of the myocardium is impaired. Nevertheless, in patients with high arterial pressure (as in this case), parenteral administration of sodium nitroprusside or trimethaphan camsylate provides moment-to-moment control of pressure. These agents are particularly well indicated for these emergent considerations since they provide moment-to-moment control of arterial pressure and permits reduction of infusion usage when pressure may need to be elevated.

ECLAMPSIA

While less commonly encountered today in medical practice, eclampsia still is an important and treatable hypertensive emergency which can prevent two deaths in each instant, that of the mother and of the infant. The disease is associated with (a) a markedly elevated arterial pressure, (b) sensory and motor neurological findings including convulsions, and (c) proteinuria during the third stage of labor. Reduction of arterial pressure will prevent the severe clinical symptoms; and delivery of the baby will result in cure of the problem. It is clear that following delivery, reduction of the severely elevated pressure will ensue and the acute problem will be resolved. However, it is important for the physician to follow the patient carefully for later elevation of arterial pressure assessment for the possibility of underlying secondary forms of hypertension and, more commonly, for underlying renal disease or essential hypertension.

As indicated in Table 9.3, the treatment of choice is the intravenous infusion of rapidly acting depressor agents. Magnesium sulfate, administered in a slowly but directly administered intravenous injection, has been used for decades as an effective means of reducing arterial pressure and convulsions. Cryptenamine, also an old agent, has been effective but is less used today. This is one of the veratrum alkaloids that can be administered by intravenous infusion and is very effective. However, this agent may be associated with nausea and vomiting. Nitroprusside sodium is also effective, but it should not be administered for prolonged time periods because of the potential of thiocyanate toxicity not only to the mother but also to the fetus. If used, thiocyanate levels should be carefully monitored.

Table 9.4. Eclampsia

Df:	Severely elevated blood pressure with convulsions in final stages of labor
Rx:	• Magnesium SO_4 (iv)
	• Cryptenamine (iv)
	• Nitroprusside sodium (iv)
	• Immediate delivery of the baby

One agent that should not be given to the patient with eclampsia is diozoxide. This is a potent and rapidly acting smooth muscle vasorelaxant that dilates arterioles and reduces arterial pressure. However, this agent also has the ability to relax uterine smooth muscle and thereby arrest labor, perpetuating the eclamptic process.

In the final analysis, the best treatment is the prompt and immediate delivery of the baby while also effectively controlling arterial pressure.

ACUTE OR CHRONIC RENAL FAILURE

Hypertension frequently complicates the development of acute or chronic renal failure. The rise in pressure is usually associated with intravascular volume expansion, particularly in the patient who was normotensive prior to the development of renal insufficiency. Hence, the most effective treatment is contraction of intravascular volume; however, this effort is usually thwarted by the inability of the kidneys to excrete the excess volume following the administration of a diuretic. Under these circumstances, the best form of therapy is the institution of hemodialysis until the acute renal failure is resolved or until other effective antihypertensive therapy results.

This problem is particularly important in children with acute renal failure resulting from acute poststreptococcal glomerulonephritis or other forms of acute renal insufficiency. In these children, the arterial pressure elevation may not be nearly as severe as in the adult. Thus, the elevated pressure in a pediatric patient with acute glomerulonephritis and anuria may be severe even for 160 mmHg or more systolic and 100 to 110 mmHg diastolic. Under this circumstance, it is important to seek nephrological consultation for the consideration of instituting dialysis therapy. Once the anuria is reversed and diuresis ensues, it may not be necessary to pharmacologically reduce and control arterial pressure.

In any event, once the acute renal failure is reversed, the patient should be followed carefully for the potential for later development of chronic arterial hypertension associated with chronic renal disease. (For additional discussion the reader is referred to Chapter 8.)

SUMMARY

In contrast to the frustrations encountered in the earlier years of antihypertensive therapy, a wide variety of agents are now available. No longer do we think of reducing arterial pressure for the treatment of the hypertensive emergency. We now are aware of a tremendous variety of hypertensive emergencies having a multiplicity of pressor mechanisms that may participate in the specific emergency. It is now possible to select the specific depressor agent for the treatment of the emergent situation by wedding the depressor mechanism of the drug with the pressor agent of the disease.

ANNOTATED BIBLIOGRAPHY

General references on hypertensive emergencies
1. The Joint National Committee on Detection, Evaluation, and Treatment of High Blood Pressure: The Fifth Report of the Joint National Committee on Detection, Evaluation, and Treatment of High Blood Pressure (JNC-V). *Arch Intern Med* 1993;153:154–183.

2. The Sixth Report of the Joint National Committee on Prevention, Detection, Evaluation, and Treatment of High Blood Pressure. *Arch Intern Med* 1997; 157:2413–2446.
3. Page IH, Corcoran AC, Dustan HP, Koppanyi T: Cardiovascular actions of sodium nitroprusside in animals and hypertensive patients. *Circulation* 1955;11:188.
4. Palmer RF, Lasseter KC: Sodium nitroprusside. *N Engl J Med* 1975;292:294–297.
5. Bhatia S, Frohlich ED: Hemodynamic comparison of agents useful in hypertensive emergencies. *Am Heart J* 1973;85:367–373.
6. Ledingham JGG. Management of hypertensive crises. *Hypertension* 1983;5 (Suppl III):114–119.
7. Calhoun DA, Oparil S. Treatment of hypertensive crisis. *N Engl J Med* 1990;323:1177–1183.
8. Gifford RW. Management of hypertensive crises. *JAMA* 1991;266:829–835.
9. Frohlich ED, Apstein C, Chobanian AV, Devereux RB, Dustan HP, Dzau V, et al: The heart in hypertension. *N Engl J Med* 1992;327:998–1008.
   References concerning stroke and hypertension:
10. Phillips SJ, Whisnant JP: On behalf of the National High Blood Pressure Education Program. Hypertension and the brain. *Arch Intern Med* 1992;152:938–945.
11. Wolf PA, Kannel WB, Verter J: Current status of risk factors for stroke. *Neurol Clin* 1983;1:317–343.
12. Schievink WI: Intracranial aneurysms. *N Engl J Med* 1977;336:28–40.
13. Charcot JM, Bouchard CH: Nouvelles recherches sur la pathogénie de l'hémorragie cérébrale. *Arch Physiol Norm Pathol* 1868;1:110–127, 643–665, 725–735.
14. Strandgaard S: Autoregulation of cerebral blood flow in hypertensive patients. The modifying influence of prolonged antihypertensive treatment on the tolerance to acute, drug-induced hypotension. *Circulation* 1976;53:720–727.
15. Fujii K, Weno BL, Baumbach GL, Heistad DD: Effect of antihypertensive treatment on focal cerebral infarction. *Hypertension* 1992;19:713–716.
16. The American Nimodipine Study Group. Clinical trial of nimodipine in acute ischemic stroke. *Stroke* 1992;23:3–8.
   References concerned with accelerated and malignant hypertension and its treatment:
17. Schottstaedt MF, Sokolow M. The natural history and course of hypertension with papiloedema (malignant hypertension). *Am Heart J* 1953;45:331–362.
18. Dustan HP, Schneckloth RE, Corcoran AC, Page IH: The effectiveness of long-term treatment of malignant hypertension. *Circulation* 1958;18:644–651.
19. Kincaid-Smith P, McMichael J, Murphy EA. The clinical course and pathology of hypertension with papilloedema (malignant hypertension). *Q J Med* 1958;27:117–153.
20. Wrong O: Retinal changes in malignant/accelerated hypertension. *BMJ* 1986; 1:483.
21. Bing RF, Heagerty AM, Russell GI, Swales DJ, Thurston H. Prognosis in malignant hypertension. *J Hypertens* 1986;4(Suppl 6):S42–S44.
22. Kincaid-Smith P. Malignant hypertension. *J Hypertens* 1991;9:893–899.
23. Gavras H, Oliver N, Aitchison J, Begg C, Briggs JD, Brown JJ, et al: Abnormalities of coagulation and the development of malignant phase hypertension. *Kidney Int* 1975;8:S252–S261.
24. Nicholls K, Walker RG, Dowling JP, Kincaid-Smith P: Malignant IgA nephropathy. *Am J Kidney Dis* 1985;5:42–46.

25. Lim KG, Isles CG, Hodsman GP, Lever AF, Robertson JWK. Malignant hypertension in women of childbearing age and its relation to the oral contraceptive pill. *BMJ* 1987;1:1057–1059.
26. Sevitt LH, Evans DJ, Wrong OM. Acute oliguric renal failure due to accelerated (malignant) hypertension. *Q J Med* 1971;40:127–144.
27. Isles CG, McLay A, Boulton-Jones JM. Recovery in malignant hypertension presenting as acute renal failure. *Q J Med* 1984;53:439–452.
28. Ledingham JCG, Rajagopalan B. Cerebral complications in the treatment of accelerated hypertension. *Q J Med* 1979;48:25–41.
   References dealing with hypertensive encephalopathy
29. Dinsdale HB: Hypertensive encephalopathy. *Stroke* 1982;13:717–719.
30. Healton EB, Brust JC, Feinfield DA, Thomson GE. Hypertensive encephalopathy and the neurological manifestations of malignant hypertension. *Neurology* 1982;32:127–132.
31. Strandgaard S, Paulson OB. Cerebral autoregulation. *Stroke* 1984;15:414–416.
32. Lassen NA, Agnoli A. The upper limit of autoregulation of cerebral blood flow: On the pathogenesis of hypertensive encephalopathy. *Scand J Clin Lab Invest* 1972;30:113–116.
   References focused on dissecting aortic aneurysm and its treatment
33. Larson EW, Edwards WD. Risk factors for aortic dissection: a necropsy study of 161 cases. *Am J Cardiol* 1984;53:849–855.
34. Slater EE, DeSanctis RW. The clinical recognition of dissecting aortic aneurysm. *Am J Med* 1976;60:625–633.
35. Wheat MW. Acute dissecting aneurysm of the aorta: diagnosis and treatment—1979. *Am Heart J* 1989;99:854–862.
36. Granto DE, Dee P, Gibson RS. Utility of two-dimensional echocardiography in suspected ascending aortic dissection. *Am J Cardio* 1985;56:123–129.
37. Mugge A, Daniel WG, Laas J, Grote R, Lichtlen PR. False negative diagnosis of proximal aortic dissection by computerised tomography or angiography and possible explanations based on transoesophageal echocardiographic findings. *Am J Cardiol* 1990;65:527–528.
   References dealing with pheochromocytoma and catecholamine excess syndromes
38. Manger WM, Gifford RW, Jr: *Clinical and Experimental Pheochromocytoma,* 2nd edition. Blackwell Science, Cambridge, 1996, 570 pp.
39. Sjoerdsma A, Engelman K, Waldmann TA, Cooperman LN, Hammond NG. Pheochromocytoma: Current concepts of diagnosis and treatment. *Ann Intern Med* 1966;65:1302–1326.
40. Manger WM, Gifford RW Jr. Current concepts of pheochromocytoma. *Cardiovasc Med* 1975;3:289–303.
41. Bravo EL, Tarazi RC, Fouad FM, Textor SC, Gifford RW Jr, Vidt DG. Blood pressure regulation in pheochromocytoma. *Hypertension* 1982;4(Suppl II):II193–II199.
42. Bravo EL, Tarazi RC, Fouad FM, Vidt DG, Gifford RW Jr. Clonidine-suppression test: A useful aid in the diagnosis of pheochromocytoma. *N Engl J Med* 1981;305:623–626.

Chapter 10

Other Clinical Considerations: Special Populations

SPECIAL POPULATIONS

About 30 years ago, we initiated a series of clinical studies at the University of Oklahoma that were designed to identify pathophysiological characteristics of patients with essential hypertension with respect to well-defined clinical, demographic, and physiological subgroupings. The goal of this overall effort was to determine whether there would be a potential therapeutic benefit of wedding the operative pathophysiological operating mechanisms in these patients with mechanisms of actions of antihypertensive drug classes. In doing so, we envisioned that it might be possible to provide a more enlightened approach to antihypertensive therapy and the overall management of patients with hypertension. As with most efforts of this nature, some findings were applicable whereas others were not.

Thus, initially, in the latter 1960s, while still on the staff of the Cleveland Clinic research division, we identified a group of patients having clinical complaints associated with hyperdynamic, hemodynamic circulatory characteristics, and increased responsiveness to beta-adrenergic receptor agonists and antagonists. Some of these patients had borderline and even sustained essential hypertension. We subsequently identified important hemodynamic differences between younger and older patients with isolated systolic hypertension. The younger patients with isolated systolic hypertension demonstrated hemodynamically an elevated cardiac output whereas the older patients had an increased total peripheral resistance. This supported earlier findings that a beta-adrenergic receptor blocking agent might be useful in the younger patients, and that a diuretic drug or other agents might be useful in the older patients.

Having been heartened by these early clinical experiences, we then began a series of studies at the University of Oklahoma in which we compared the physiological characteristics of black and white patients with essential hypertension. Later, after establishing our clinical research program in New Orleans at the Ochsner Institutions, we continued these comparisons of patients with respect to race. These studies were followed by other efforts in which we compared patients who were lean or obese, younger or older, and with and without target organ involvement of the heart or kidney. The following discussions summarize these and other findings that support the merits supporting the concept that antihypertensive treatment may be assisted by specific clinical and demographic identifiers. Clearly, this discussion reflects my personal thoughts on each area supported by our personal clinical investigative efforts and publications. In most of these subject areas they are consistent with the national educational reports, consensus, and health outcome findings.

BORDERLINE HYPERTENSIONS

Hyperdynamic Beta-Adrenergic Circulatory State

As already discussed more extensively (Chapter 6), patients with hypertension may be identified clinically and hemodynamically with respect to clinical and physiological characteristics that suggest a hyperdynamic circulation. We were encouraged by our findings since this became the first clinically identifiable group of patients that we could identify having a specific clinical syndrome lending itself to characterization physiologically and to specific antihypertensive therapy. Thus, Doctors Harriet Dustan, Robert Tarazi, Irvine Page, and myself became aware of a specific group of patients with complaints of rapid and forceful cardiac action that was associated with disturbing palpitations, ectopic cardiac beats, symptoms of cutaneous flushing, sweating, an exaggerated increase in heart rate when assuming upright posture, and intense anxiety (if not frank hysteria) that was associated with an exaggerated rapid heart action.

Physiologically, their hemodynamic findings were those of a hyperdynamic circulation manifested by a faster heart rate, elevated cardiac output, and increased myocardial contractility. Moreover, when some of these patients were subjected to an isoproterenol infusion, there was an exaggerated response of heart rate and a provocation of their clinical symptoms and other complaints reported on their clinical presentation. Subsequently, we documented an idiopathic mitral valve prolapse syndrome in these patients that was also associated with increase serum catecholamine (i.e., norepinephrine) levels. Moreover, when these patients were treated with a beta-adrenergic receptor blocking agent, their symptoms remitted, the elevated arterial pressure was reduced, and the evidence of their hyperdynamic hemodynamic indices were normalized.

Thus, it seemed to us that these patients with hypertension were likely to benefit from a prescribed beta-adrenergic receptor blocking drug. Such treatment continues to be advised for these patients with the hyperdynamic beta-adrenergic circulatory state. It not only normalizes the arterial pressure, but relieves the symptoms associated with the hyperdynamic circulation and the increased beta-adrenergically mediated complaints.

Borderline Hypertension

Some of the foregoing groups of patients could be characterized as having normal diastolic pressure (less than 90 mmHg) at some times, but at other times their pressures were elevated (above 90 mmHg). (More recently, these patients may be characterized as having systolic pressures ranging from 140 through 159 mmHg.) At the time that these patients were initially identified as being a potentially different class of patients with hypertension (in the 1960s), they were said to have "labile hypertension" because of the impressive variability of their diastolic pressures. However, it soon became apparent that the arterial pressure of all patients with systemic hypertension had extremely variable or "labile" pressures. For this reason, the diagnosis of "labile hypertension" was discontinued and the term "borderline hypertension" was introduced by those of us interested in this problem. Unfortunately, our epidemiologically oriented colleagues had also introduced the term of borderline hypertension. They referred to those patients with hypertension whose systolic pressures ranged from 140 to 159 mmHg and/or with diastolic pressures ranging from 90 to 94 mmHg. This term had been chosen by our epidemiologically oriented colleagues to suggest that this was a group of patients whose overall cardiovascular risk was neither that of the normal population (less than 140 mmHg systolic and/or 90 mmHg diastolic), nor as great as those patients with established hypertension whose systolic and diastolic pressures were greater than 159 and/or 94 mmHg, respectively.

As suggested earlier, younger patients having borderline (diastolic) hypertension (as we described for the physiological studies) had an elevated cardiac output, a faster heart rate, and increased myocardial contractility (see Chapter 1). Unlike the other patients who had a hyperdynamic beta-adrenergic circulatory state, however, these patients with "borderline hypertension" demonstrated normal cardiac responsiveness to an intravenous isoproterenol infusion. These findings were confirmed by a number of other clinical investigative groups studying this problem. Moreover, it was learned subsequently that their elevated cardiac output eventually declined with time as total peripheral resistance increased (even though their heart rate remained faster) as a sustained state of blood pressure elevation was established. Thus, over a number of years, when these patients had been followed longitudinally in an impressive study by Per Lund-Johansen and his colleagues in Oslo, the hyperkinetic circulation documented 20 years earlier was converted to a hemodynamic pattern of normal cardiac output and increased total peripheral resistance (as their hemodynamic measurements were repeated after 10 and, then again, after 20 years).

Thus, the state of sustained essential hypertension in these patients could be attributed to a normalization of cardiac output and an increased total peripheral resistance that was more or less uniformly distributed throughout the component organ circulations. As indicated above, these patients with hypertension did not demonstrate increased responsiveness to the intravenous beta-adrenergic receptor agonist when their earlier stages of hypertension was associated with a hyperdynamic circulation. Nevertheless, they did seem to respond well to beta-adrenergic blocking therapy alone or in combination with a thiazide diuretic.

The therapeutic approach to these patients today may be quite variable depending upon the associated clinical circumstances. Thus, if the pressure does vary from the normotensive to hypertensive pressures, it may be wise to simply monitor the patient's pressures with home measurements and periodically in the office. Indeed, if their pressures remain less than 140 and 90 mmHg, systolic and diastolic, respectively, and there is no history of premature death in the family, no evidence of target organ involvement by clinical and laboratory studies, and no other cardiovascular risk factors, it might be wise to continue to follow the patient without prescribing any antihypertensive therapy other than the very reasonable recommendations for lifestyle modification. These recommendations would include weight control, sodium restriction, smoke cessation, alcohol moderation, and a regular program of isotonic exercise (see Chapter 3). Some of these patients have also been termed as having variously "white coat hypertension," "hyperreactors," etc. However, if there is a strong family history of premature cardiovascular death and morbidity, and particularly if there are lines of clinical evidence to suggest early target organ involvement, I, personally, would institute a program of antihypertensive therapy. Indeed, this thinking is consistent with the current recommendations in the JNC-VI report. I believe that this would be particularly justified if the office systolic or diastolic pressures consistently exceeded 140 and 89 mmHg, respectively. At the present time, however, there are less compelling reasons for instituting antihypertensive pharmacological therapy in those patients without risk factors or target involvement and with so-called isolated borderline systolic hypertension. These individuals with systolic pressures, falling between 140 and 159 mmHg (and with diastolic pressures less than 90 mmHg), have not been shown by prospective clinical trials to demonstrate reduced cardiovascular morbidity and mortality with specific antihypertensive therapy. Such a controlled multicenter, clinical trial is being planned for implementation in the very near future. The results of this (and confirmatory studies) will resolve all existing questions concerning pressures in excess of 139 and 89 mmHg, respectively.

AGE CONSIDERATIONS

In this age of evidence-based medicine there is, perhaps, no area recommending antihypertensive treatment that is better supported than there is for the treatment of the elderly patient with hypertension. This is particularly fortunate since this is the one area of the general population in the United States (and, for that matter, in most industrialized societies) that is growing tremendously. Thus, individuals who are 65 years of age of older account for over 15% of the overall population, a figure which no doubt will continue to increase over the near future into the beginning of the 21st century. Not only is this a significant population that is at increased risk for cardiovascular diseases and their complications, but more than 50 % of these people have an abnormally elevated systolic and/or diastolic pressure. Newer terminology has crept into the literature that refer not only to the elderly, but to the "old elderly" and the "old, old elderly," referring to the growing numbers of people who are now in their 80s, 90s, and even over 100 years of age. This strikingly high (and increasing) percentage of people in the general population includes patients with isolated systolic hypertension, a segment of the hypertensive population which has been shown clearly to benefit from antihypertensive drug therapy. The recent JNC-V and JNC-VI reports have repeatedly emphasized that hypertension occurs in about 60%, 71%, and 61% of non-Hispanic whites, non-Hispanic blacks, and Mexican-Americans, respectively. Indeed, the recent working group on "Hypertension in the Elderly" of the National High Blood Pressure Education Program cited Census Bureau data in the United States that estimates over 3.2 million Americans were 85 years and older in 1990; and that by 2050, there will be more than 16 million Americans who will be older than 85 years of age.

In these elderly patients with hypertension (whether diastolic or isolated systolic), cardiac output is either normal or reduced depending upon the degree of left ventricular hypertrophy and the extent of other cardiac complications including epicardial atherosclerotic coronary arterial disease, obesity, diabetes mellitus, and other comorbid problems. Thus, not only does the increased total peripheral resistance play a major role in the hemodynamic alterations of the disease but, because of the reduced compliance and distensibility of the aorta and larger arteries with advancing age and atherosclerosis, the increased impedance imposed upon the left ventricle is further exacerbated (Figure 10.1).

Each of these vascular factors only serve to elevate the systolic pressure and the metabolic demands imposed upon the left ventricle. Moreover, since the major determinant of myocardial oxygen consumption is the tension of the left ventricular chamber (which, in turn, is directly dependent upon the height of systolic pressure

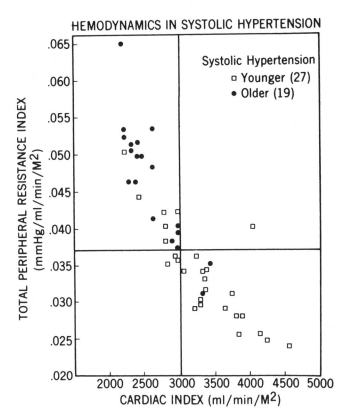

Figure 10.1. Presentation of cardiac index and total peripheral resistance in patients with systolic hypertension. Note that older patients (greater than 65 years old) have a higher total peripheral resistance and lower cardiac output than younger patients with isolated systolic hypertension (Reprinted with permission from Adamopoulos PN, Chrysanthakopoulis SG, Frohlich ED: Systolic hypertension: Non-homogeneous diseases. *Am J Cardiol* 36:697–701, 1975.)

and its transverse diameter) the cardiac complications are all the more meaningful. Finally, since these factors all impact upon the need for systemic perfusion by a heart that is progressively more challenged by the disease, is there any small wonder why cardiac failure is the most common cause of hospitalization in the United States today? Add to the hemodynamic factor the increased collagen in the ventricle of the older individual and in the myocardium of the patient with ischemia, the pathophysiological p. 185 reasoning for the rise in cardiac failure becomes clear. To this end, the most recent data from the Framingham Heart Study confirms its earlier report of the 1960s that demonstrated hypertension to be the most common cause of cardiac failure in the United States today; the second most common cause is hypertension complicated by atherosclerotic (ischemic) heart disease.

As cardiac involvement becomes more evident, cardiac output progressively declines and, pari passu, so does its distribution to the organ circulations. Thus, renal blood flow diminishes with advancing age and, with it, glomerular filtration rate and the renal filtration fraction. Nephrosclerosis is a major renal complication that is a feature of the aging patient without hypertension; and this is even more evident in the patient with hypertension, diabetes mellitus, or who is black. We can, therefore, clearly understand why end-stage renal disease continues to rise in this country despite the increasing numbers of patients receiving antihypertensive drug therapy. These changes in organ blood flow and function are also evident in other circulations including the splanchnic with its inherent implications on hepatic function and the metabolism of naturally occurring humoral and hormonal agents as well as of exogenously administered drugs, electrolytes, and other chemicals.

As already indicated, recommendations for antihypertensive treatment programs have now advanced. Earlier reports were consensus documents whereas they now rely more upon evidence-based medicine. In no place is this more clear-cut than in the recent JNC-VI report and recommendations. It is indeed fortunate that, in this age of increasing impact reliance by Medicare and health maintenance organizations, these evidence based therapeutic guidelines provide a clinical reasoning for antihypertensive treatment guidelines directed toward the elderly. Thus, the statements in JNC-V and JNC-VI of the diuretic and beta-adrenergic receptor blocking drugs (and possibly certain calcium antagonists) are recommended for their initial therapy because controlled, multicenter trials have demonstrated the reduced morbidity and mortality that were associated with these agents.

We have already referred to an impressive meta-analysis of Thijs and associates, which confirmed the concept that treatment of elderly patients with hypertension with diuretics and beta-blockers will reduce morbidity and mortality from stroke and coronary heart disease (Chapter 7). The earlier meta-analysis of Collins et al, predicted that diuretic and beta-blocker therapy would reduce deaths from strokes and coronary heart disease by 40 to 45% and 20 to 25%, respectively. Both disease outcomes were significantly decreased, stroke by 43% but coronary heart disease by only 14% (the latter still statistically significant). However, in the former (and more recent meta-analysis) by Thijs et al, in which hydrochlorothiazide was employed in much lower doses (25 to 50 mg rather than 100 mg in the former meta-analysis), the prediction of reduction of deaths from strokes was reaffirmed and the reduction of deaths from coronary heart disease of 26% was fully affirmed. Supporting these recommendations of diuretics and beta-blocking agents for initial therapy, were the findings from several other multicenter trials. Thus, the European Working Party on High Blood Pressure in the Elderly Trial (EUWPHE) demonstrated, in elderly patients with diastolic hypertension (i.e., $\geq$ 95 mmHg), using a double-blinded, placebo-controlled multicenter trial with methyldopa and triamterene combined with a thiazide, the control of arterial pressure was associated with diminished mortality from strokes and coronary heart disease (and other events). More recently, another European multicenter drug trial using the calcium antagonist nitrendipine (not available in the United States) alone or with enalapril or a thiazide also demonstrated reduction in deaths from stroke. Still another less well designed study, the STONE Trial in China, strongly suggested that the long-acting formulation of the calcium antagonist nifedipine demonstrated reduction from stroke. Furthermore, in several major multicenter trials involving primarily normotensive elderly patients with coronary heart disease (following myocardial infarction or with chronic congestive heart failure), long-term treatment with a variety of ACE inhibitors demonstrated reduced mortality from coronary heart disease and cardiac failure. Finally, the (isolated) Systolic Hypertension in the Elderly Program trial (SHEP) demonstrated that elderly patients with isolated systolic hypertension had significantly reduced mortality from strokes and morbidity from strokes and coronary heart disease with diuretics and beta-blockers. This study was subsequently confirmed by the MRC Trial (from Great Britain) and the STOP Hypertension Trial (from Sweden) using similar antihypertensive agents in patients with isolated systolic hypertension.

It is perhaps worth repeating (in this chapter) the point made elsewhere in this volume that most of the foregoing drug trials so convincingly demonstrated reduction of deaths from stroke and (initially, less convincingly to some) coronary heart disease that the studies were discontinued by their respective monitoring committees. The cerebral circulation is more sensitive to the effect of arterial pressure reduction than other circulations; and, more important, when the reduction of deaths from stroke was demonstrated to the ethics and safety boards of these blinded studies, the trials were, *per force,* discontinued. Consequently, the more complex circulations (i.e., coronary and renal) required either more prolonged treatment or other studies using different treatment populations.

Nevertheless, the recommendations are very clear and much less controversial today: long-term antihypertensive therapy should now be recommended for all patients, young or elderly, with diastolic or isolated systolic hypertension. With such antihypertensive treatment programs it may now be asserted that reduction in cardiovascular morbidity and mortality will be forthcoming. The major proviso, of course, is that these patients must first be detected and evaluated and brought into a meaningful treatment program.

RACIAL CONSIDERATIONS

Epidemiological studies have repeatedly demonstrated a greater prevalence of hypertensive disease and its complications is in the black population than in the white. Thus, not only is the disease more commonly encountered in the black patient, but there is a greater likelihood that the hypertension in the black patient has a greater chance of producing target organ involvement with respect to stroke, malignant hypertension, coronary heart disease, cardiac failure, and renal functional impairment with consequent end-stage renal disease than the white patient. Therefore, hypertensive disease is considered to run a far more severe course in patients of the black race than in the white. Add to this the fact that obesity as well as diabetes mellitus is also more commonly encountered in the black, there is increasing concern and necessity for early detection and maintained treatment of their hypertension.

At present, there is no adequate explanation for the foregoing epidemiological and clinical findings. However, in our earlier studies we compared certain physiological and hemodynamic characteristics of black and white patients with stable essential hypertension whose arterial pressures, ages, gender, and body mass had been carefully matched. The results of these studies revealed that, whereas both racial groups demonstrate a decrease in their intravascular (i.e., plasma) volume as arterial pressure increased, the contraction of plasma volume was greater in those patients who were white. Moreover, plasma renin activity, which increases as plasma volume contracts, was lower (or more suppressed) in the black patients. Thus, in general, the plasma volume in the black is relatively expanded (or less contracted) as compared with the white patients with elevated arterial pressure of the same magnitude. Moreover, as arterial pressure increased in black patients, their plasma volume contracted less and their plasma renin activity was proportionately suppressed. However, plasma volume was not expanded in the black patient with hypertension as has been inaccurately interpreted from our clinical research findings; it is less contracted than in hypertensive patients who are white.

Our subsequent hemodynamic studies demonstrated that the left ventricular hypertrophy in black patients with hypertension was more closely associated with their elevated arterial pressure and total peripheral resistance than in white patients whose arterial pressures were of the same degree of elevation. Moreover, we also found that the increased renal vascular resistance in the black patient with hypertension was more closely related to the increased arterial pressure and total peripheral resistance than in the white patient whose arterial pressure of the same magnitude of elevation (Figure 10.2).

We were encouraged by the above early hemodynamic findings from our laboratory that were elucidated almost contemporaneously with the results of one of the Veterans Administration Cooperative Studies that had reported the initial findings that antihypertensive therapy reduced cardiovascular morbidity and mortality. This subsequent study demonstrated that white patients responded to antihypertensive treatment with a beta-adrenergic blocking drug (i.e., propranolol) better than black patients when these agents were employed as monotherapy. However, in that same study, when a diuretic was added to the beta-blocker, no differences between the two racial groups were evident. Subsequent studies (in yet another VA Cooperative Study) indicated that black patients seemed to be more responsive to therapy with a calcium antagonist (i.e., diltiazem). It is of particular interest for us to recall (from Chapter 4)

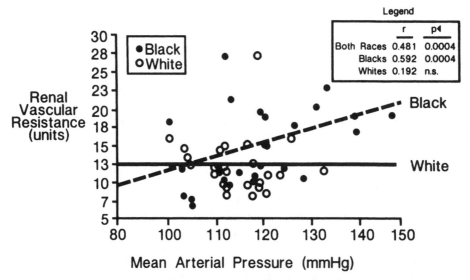

Figure 10.2. Relationship between renal vascular resistance and mean arterial pressure in black and white patients with essential hypertension. Note that there is a significant correlation between these two indices in the black patients but not the white (Reprinted with permission from Frohlich ED, Messerli FH, Dunn FG, et al: Greater renal vascular involvement in the black patient with essential hypertension. A comparison of systemic and renal hemodynamics in black and white patients. *Mineral Electrolyte Metab* 10:173–177, 1984.)

that, in addition to producing arteriolar vasodilation, the calcium antagonists also promote natriuresis (as a result of their additional action of inhibiting renal sodium-for-calcium exchange). Hence, this additional effect of the calcium antagonists on the renal tubule may provide an additional natriuretic action in patients with a more volume-dependent mechanism participating in their hypertensive disease.

Thus, even though our understanding of the differences in the pathophysiology of the hypertension in black and white patients are far from complete, there is good physiological support for arriving at some therapeutic concepts at this time. We also know that the diuretic is an excellent choice for initial monotherapy for patients of both races; but beta-blocker monotherapy for the white patient appears to be more efficacious. For this reason, the diuretic may be the wiser selection for initial therapy in the black patient with hypertension; and, should the initially selected agent be inadequate for control of pressure in either racial group, the combination of the diuretic and the beta-blocker seems to be a wise secondary selection. On the other hand, if the beta-blocker, cannot be used in the black patient, the calcium antagonist is a reasonable choice for initial therapy, particularly if the patient has more severe hypertension, angina pectoris, or any other condition that would indicate that the calcium antagonist is a wiser choice. Even though the black patient may not respond as well to the ACE inhibitors (or, for that matter, an angiotensin II, type I, receptor antagonist) as the white patient with hypertension, it might be wise to select an ACE inhibitor for initial therapy particularly if that patient has diabetes mellitus, proteinuria, or renal functional impairment. However, if that patient does not demonstrate adequate control of arterial pressure with that ACE inhibitor in maximal doses), it might be worthwhile to maintain treatment with that agent (perhaps in a lower dose), and add to it an agent from one of the other antihypertensive drug classes (i.e., a diuretic, calcium antagonist, or an alpha-beta receptor blocker). With demonstrated control of pressure it might be worthwhile and, perhaps, more cost-effective to prescribe a single tablet containing the ACE inhibitor (or angiotensin II receptor (type 1) antagonist) with a diuretic or a calcium antagonist. Indeed, as suggested in JNC-VI, tablets of combination therapy may be a wise choice, particularly since newer combinations and wiser dosing selections are now available.

GENDER

In general, the prevalence of hypertension among men and women are about the same. However, most epidemiological studies have indicated that complications from hypertensive cardiac and vascular disease appears to be less frequent and severe among women until they reach the age of menopause or even a little later. However, after that age the morbidity and mortality from hypertension and its cardiovascular complications seems to catch up in the female gender. Notwithstanding, at any age, systolic and diastolic pressures are higher in black women than white.

With respect to specific therapeutic recommendations in women than in men, there are several points that are worth noting. First, the early multicenter antihypertensive drug trials did not include as great a percentage of female patients than of men. In part, this may have been because of less consciousness of the necessity to include patients of both genders; but, there were other considerations including the lack of inclusion of "females of child-bearing potential" in new drug trials because of concerns of potential teratogenicity in the unborn child. However, at this point, most authorities presently believe that when blood pressure is elevated in women it should be treated as vigorously as in men. This concept is expressed in all JNC reports. Moreover, since there is evidence that women have greater acuity of health concerns than men and, when they receive drug treatment, their adherence to antihypertensive treatment programs may even be better than in men. This consideration is true not only with respect to pharmacotherapy, but also with the use of lifestyle modifications using non-drug therapies.

In any event, the more recent long-term clinical antihypertensive drug trials that have included large numbers of women have not demonstrated any major gender differences in the response of arterial pressure to the various antihypertensive agents and in the health care outcomes of treatment. This concept has been emphasized in both of the more recent JNC reports. Nevertheless, their are certain considerations concerning selection of drugs for women that merit consideration. First, in the premenopausal women who finds it necessary to take diuretics for fluid retention during the menstrual cycle, it might be wise to select diuretics for initial treatment in the less than full doses. Then, if arterial pressure (or the fluid retention) is not adequately controlled, an increase to full dosage would be indicated, taking particular care to protect the patient from potential hypokalemia and other metabolic side effects. Second, if the patient requires aspirin (other non-steroidal anti-inflammatory drugs) for pain or discomfort, the patient should be advised that these drugs may inhibit the antihypertensive effectiveness of the diuretics and/or other antihypertensive agents. In that case, the physician should prescribe agents to relieve pain that do not operate through the mechanism of inhibition of prostaglandin synthetase (e.g., acetaminophen). Thirdly, if a premenopausal woman elects to initiate oral contraceptive therapy, it is worth remembering that hypertension is more frequent in the woman taking oral contraceptives (especially if she is older, obese, or has diabetes mellitus). More generally, blood pressure is higher in a group of women who use oral contraceptives than those who do not. It is fair to say, however, that the oral contraceptive is not contraindicated in women who have hypertension or have "high normal" pressures; but it is likewise worthy to remember that any patient who uses an oral contraceptive agent, should have her blood pressure taken periodically during such treatment (particularly at the outset).

In general, I usually check the patient's blood pressure after 1 and 3 months and then every 3 or 4 months. One way to obviate frequent returns to the physician's office for blood pressure checks is to advise the patient to have her own sphygmomanometer at home and to keep a record of her pressures. I usually advise against an electronic device since they usually cannot be properly calibrated. Then, if the measured pressures demonstrate a consistent rise or if they reach "hypertensive levels," I advise the patients to report this to me at their earliest concern. If blood pressures reach elevated levels, the doses of estrogen and progestogen may be reduced, pressures should continue to be monitored and, if pressure continues to remain elevated, another form of contraception should be advised.

Alternately, it may be wise to prescribe an antihypertensive agent. Following the same line of thinking, some word may be appropriate about advising the use of estrogen replacement therapy in postmenopausal women. There may be a rise of arterial pressure associated with the use of this important preventive medical approach to ischemic heart disease, osteoporosis, and other diseases. However, under these circumstances, I usually advise these patients to follow the same line of home blood pressure monitoring with records and to advise me if there is concern about blood pressure increases or development of hypertensive levels of arterial pressure. In the "high risk" patient, antihypertensive therapy may be necessary.

A word might be in order concerning hypertension in **pregnancy**. If the patient has had an elevated blood pressure prior to any pregnancy (termed "chronic hypertension" in the JNC advisory reports), they may remain on the same drug therapy (including diuretics and most all other antihypertensive drugs) during their pregnancies with the exception of ACE inhibitors and angiotensin II (type I) receptor antagonists which are definitely contraindicated in the pregnant woman. On the other hand, if the patient develops hypertension during pregnancy, most obstetricians are concerned about the use of diuretics and, under that circumstance, they prescribe hydralazine, methyldopa, and beta-adrenergic receptor blocking agents. Although not written about extensively and not included in general recommendations, I have found that certain long-acting calcium antagonists have been very useful, particularly in the hypertensive and preeclamptic patient who cannot take the other medications because of side effects or other contraindications (e.g., asthma, past history of hemolytic anemia with methyldopa). A recent more extensive report by the Working Group on High Blood Pressure in Pregnancy has been published by the National High Blood Pressure Education Program (Am J Obstet Gynecol 163:1689–1712, 1990) and Pediatrics 98;649–658,1996.

HYPERTENSION IN CHILDREN AND ADOLESCENTS

For years we have been taught that hypertension in children should suggest a secondary form of hypertension. Clearly, blood pressure should be taken in all children; and, in general, this may be an important admonition for the physician to search for secondary causes. However, the search for secondary causation of hypertension may not be at all rewarding and the search for the secondary cause may be expensive and frustrating, especially in the young person with a strong family history of essential hypertension. On the other hand, the demonstration of a secondary form of hypertension may be identified readily and with ease (e.g., aortic coarctation, renal arterial disease, over-the-counter drugs). Nevertheless, several points are important to bear in mind: (1) it is not at all expensive to search for the presence of femoral arterial pulsations, providing a high index for the presence of aortic coarctation; (2) it may be worthwhile to consider an adrenal causation of the hypertension if certain physical characteristics suggest this possibility (e.g, hirsutism, adrenal genitalism, evidence of acromegaly, thyroid disease, and, clearly, a strong family history of hypertension); and (3) the history of renal infections, presence of an enlarged kidney and polycythemia (i.e., possible polycystic renal disease), and renal arterial bruits (especially if there is a diastolic component to the bruit) should suggest further evaluation or consultative assistance.

I have not yet mentioned the measurement of arterial pressure in the child or adolescent patient. First and foremost, it is necessary to use the proper sphygmomanometer cuff having the appropriate width. Second, the blood pressure, if found to be elevated, should be taken (in triplicate) on at least three visits unless there is an immediate concern about an elevated pressure. Under these circumstances, the physician should, of course, follow through with the overall management of the patient. There has been much discussion on just what are the exact definitions of an elevated blood pressure in children. This issue has been of particular concern to pediatricians

Table 10.1. 95th Percentile of Blood Pressure by Selected Ages in Girls and Boys, by the 50th and 75th Height Percentiles*

Age (Years)	Girls' SBP/DBP		Boys' SBP/DBP	
	50th Percentile for Height	75th Percentile for Height	50th Percentile for Height	75th Percentile for Height
1	104/58	105/95	102/57	504/58
6	111/73	112/73	114/74	115/75
12	123/80	124/81	123/81	125/82
17	129/84	130/85	136/87	138/88

*Adapted from the report by the NHBPEP Working Group on Hypertension Control in Children and Adolescents. SBP indicates systolic blood pressure; DBP diastolic blood pressure.

who have responded to this concern with recommendation that blood pressures (the average of three measurements), if at the 95th percentile or greater is considered to be elevated (Table 10.1). The fifth Korotkoff sound (or disappearance of the sound) is now used by all pediatricians for the diastolic pressure. For further details on this subject the reader is referred to the Working Group Report on Hypertension Control in Children and Adolescents, which is an update on the 1987 task force report on high blood pressure in children and adolescents (Pediatrics 98:649–658, 1996).

OBESITY

Hyperinsulinemia.

Last, but certainly not the least, many clinical investigators have been attracted to the long-standing clinical observation of the association of hypertension, diabetes mellitus, obesity, and hyperlipidemia. The more recent studies in this sphere of clinical investigation have focused on the finding that these patients (whether black or white) require higher doses of insulin infusion to control blood sugar during a glucose infusion. This finding, termed insulin resistance associated with hyperinsulinemia, in patients with hypertension, diabetes mellitus, hyperlipidemia and obesity, suggested the hypothesis that the increased circulating blood levels of insulin might serve as an important pathophysiological (if not pathogenetic) mechanism underlying the hypertensive disease state, if not the syndrome of these associated diseases. This concept was reinforced by the experimental findings of Landsberg and Young who suggested that the increased circulating insulin levels may serve to stimulate certain areas in the hindbrain that enhance adrenergic outflow from the brain to the cardiovascular and renal systems thereby increasing arterial pressure.

This area of clinical investigation continues to be under very active investigation, is controversial, and, as yet, remains unresolved. However, it provides additional concepts for the underlying mechanism(s) of hypertension in the black patient, the overweight patient, certainly the patient with diabetes mellitus, and even the patient with hyperlipidemia. Moreover, it may also provide an important way of thinking in developing a rationale for selecting antihypertensive therapy in each of these clinical complicating factors associated with hypertension. We can think, then, of the more intense cardiac, vascular, renal, and cerebral involvement in hypertension as well as the participating mechanisms underlying the hypervolemia, hyperinsulinism and, perhaps, increase sympathetic participation in the overall clinical problem. There are several other postulated mechanisms that may also be related to the clinical pathophysiological state: increased sodium retention in the black and obese patients and the participation of certain cellular growth factors (e.g., insulin-like growth factor) that might account for the cardiac, vascular, and renal disease (Figure 10.3).

Hemodynamics

In addition to the foregoing pathophysiological considerations, early hemodynamic studies from our laboratory had demonstrated that intravascular (i.e., plasma) volume was expanded in patients who are obese. This expanded circulating volume was redistributed from the peripheral to the central circulations to increase venous return to the heart and to elevate cardiac output in the obese patients. Associated with the increased cardiac output in obese patients with hypertension is an increased renal blood flow and glomerular filtration rate. These changes may be associated with an increased glomerular filtration fraction which, in studies in experimental hypertension, has been associated with hyperfiltration, glomerulosclerosis with hypercellularity and dilated capillaries, and microalbuminuria. Since the left ventricle responds to the pressure overload of hypertension with a concentric hypertrophy and to the increased volume or preload by an eccentric hypertrophy, the ventricular overload in the obese patient with essential hypertension is more complex, requiring adaptation to both the pressure and volume overload. These findings tend to explain why there are greater renal and cardiac risks in

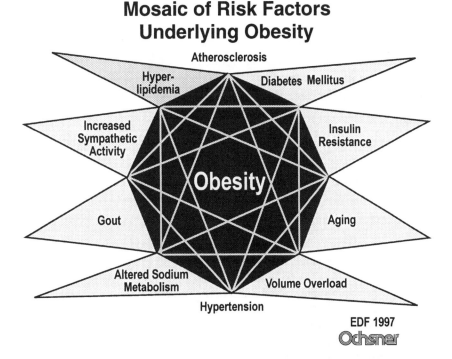

Figure 10.3. Another mosaic of factors that interrelate with one another in patients with obesity.

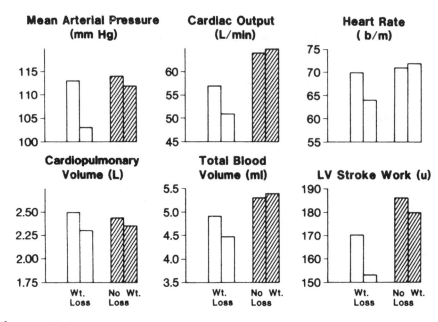

Figure 10.4. Systemic hemodynamic characteristics of obese patients. In open bars are those patients who demonstrate a weight reduction; and the cross-hatch bars represent those obese patients who failed to lose weight. (Reprinted with permission from Reisin E, Frohlich ED, Messerli FH, et al: Cardiovascular changes after weight reduction in obesity hypertension. *Ann Intern Med* 98:315–319, 1983.)

obese hypertensive patients. With weight reduction that is associated with a diminution in arterial pressure, intravascular (plasma) volume diminishes; and this is associated with a reduction in cardiopulmonary volume and cardiac output (Figure 10.4).

Management

It follows, therefore, that treatment of the obese patient with hypertension should be directed to a well-designed weight reduction program that should be worked out (most importantly) with a very practical dietician who can communicate well with the patient. It is broadly acknowledged that there is a high degree of recalcitrance with any weight reduction program; and, one of the keys to its success, is a close follow-up with the patient with clear communication. The use of a nutritional consultant or dietician may even be wise. It is important to help the patient to understand the high risk rate of premature cardiovascular death in the obese patient with multiple risk factors (e.g., obesity and hypertension which, not infrequently are associated with diabetes mellitus, hyperlipidemia, hyperuricemia and possibly gout, and not infrequently with smoking and increased alcohol intake.

The present selection of pharmacological agents directed to appetite suppression and weight reduction is an exercise in frustration for the practicing physician since most agents will also elevate arterial pressure. Other agents (such as the recent problems with "phen-phen") may be responsible for the development of cardiac valvular lesions. Most workers in this area are not disconcerted and look forward to a variety of new agents that may be useful for the obese patient with hypertension without further elevating arterial pressure. One such compound under active investigation is leptin, a recently discovered natural peptide that may suppress appetite, reduce body weight and, hopefully, arterial pressure.

For the time being, however, one of the antihypertensive agents that may be of some success in reducing pressure is the diuretic since, as described above, this agent will contract intravascular volume and thereby reduce cardiac output and arterial pressure, pari passu. Also suggested is the judicious use of the diuretic in combination with other classes of antihypertensive agents—obviously superimposed upon a meaningful weight reduction approach to diet therapy.

REFERENCES

The following references (many are personal) were selected by the author to supplement his discussion on the respective topics. These references, although many are dated, support current contentions made relative to these timely, yet (some) controversial areas.

Hyperdynamic Beta-Adrenergic Circulating State

Frohlich ED, Dustan HP, Page IH: Hyperdynamic beta-adrenergic circulatory state. *Arch Intern Med* 117:614–619, 1966.

Frohlich ED, Tarazi RC, Dustan HP: Hyperdynamic beta-adrenergic circulatory state: Increased beta receptor responsiveness. *Arch Intern Med* 123:1–7, 1969.

De Carvalho JGR, Messerli FH, Frohlich ED: Mitral valve prolapse and borderline hypertension. *Hypertension* 1:518–522, 1979.

Borderline Hypertension

Frohlich ED: Defining borderline hypertension: the problem. Blood Pressure. (in press).

Frohlich ED, Kozul VJ, Tarazi RC, et al: Physiological comparison of labile and essential hypertension. *Circ Res* 27(1):55–69, 1970.

Julius S, Schork MA: Borderline hypertension—a critical review. *J Chron Dis* 23:723–754, 1971.

Messerli FH, de Carvalho JGR, Christie B, et al: Systemic and regional hemodynamics in low, normal, and high cardiac output in borderline hypertension. *Circulation* 58:441–448, 1978.

Aging

Adamopoulos PN, Chrysanthakopoulis SG, Frohlich ED: Systolic hypertension: Nonhomogeneous diseases. *Am J Cardiol* 36:697–701, 1975.

Dahlof B, Lindholm LH, Hansson L, et al: Morbidity and mortality in the Swedish Trial in Old Patients with Hypertension (STOP-Hypertension). *Lancet* 338:1281–1285, 1991.

Frohlich ED: Hypertension in the elderly. *Curr Probl Cardiol* 13:313–367, 1988.

Frohlich ED: Hypertension in the elderly. *Cardiovasc Risk Factors* 4:127–132, 1994.

Frohlich ED, Messerli FH: Systolic hypertension in the elderly. In: Safar ME, Simon ACH, Weiss YA, eds. *Arterial and Venous Systems in Essential Hypertension.* Dordrecht, The Netherlands: Martinus Nijhoff Publishers, 1987, pp. 105–114.

Lakatta EG, Cohen JD, Fleg JL, et al: Hypertension in the elderly: Age and disease related complications and therapeutic implications. *J Cardiovasc Drug Ther* 7:643–653, 1993.

Levy D, Larson MG, Vasan RS, et al: The progression from hypertension to congestive heart failure. *JAMA* 275:1557–1562, 1996.

Messerli FH, Sundgaard-Riise K, Ventura HO, et al: Essential hypertension in the elderly: Haemodynamics, intravascular volume, plasma renin activity, and circulating catecholamines. *Lancet* 2:983–986, 1983.

MRC Working Party. Medical Research Council trial of treatment of hypertension in older adults: principal results. *Br Med J* 304:405–412, 1992.

Sagie A, Larson MG, Levy D: The natural history of borderline isolated systolic hypertension. *N Engl J Med* 329:1912–1917, 1993.

Systolic Hypertension in the Elderly Program Cooperative Research Group. (SHEP). Implications of the Systolic Hypertension in the Elderly Program. *Hypertension* 21:335–343, 1993.

Obesity

Frohlich ED: Hypertension. In: Abrams WB, Beers MH, Berkow R, eds. *The Merck Manual of Geriatrics.* 2nd ed. Whitehouse Station, NJ: Merck Research Laboratories 1995, pp. 454–474.

Frohlich ED: Obesity and hypertension: Hemodynamic aspects. *Ann Epidemiol* 1:287–293, 1991.

Frohlich ED, Messerli FH, Reisin E, et al: The problem of obesity and hypertension. *Hypertension* 5(III):71–78, 1983.

Frohlich ED, Reisin E: Hemodynamics in patients with overweight and hypertension. In: Safar ME, Fouad-Tarazi FM, eds. *The Heart in Hypertension.* The Netherlands: Kluwer Academic Publishers, 1989, pp. 105–122.

Messerli FH, Christie B, de Carvalho JGR, et al: Obesity and essential hypertension. Hemodynamics, intravascular volume, sodium excretion, and plasma renin activity. *Arch Intern Med* 141:81–85, 1981.

Messerli FH, Sundgaard-Riise K, Reisin E, et al: Dimorphic cardiac adaptation to obesity and arterial hypertension. *Ann Intern Med* 99:757–761, 1983.

Reisin E, Frohlich ED: Hemodynamics in obesity. In: Zanchetti A, Tarazi RC, eds. *Handbook of Hypertension* Vol 7. Amsterdam: Elsevier Science Publishers B.V., 1986, pp. 280–297.

Reisin E, Frohlich ED, Messerli FH, et al: Cardiovascular changes after weight reduction in obesity hypertension. *Ann Intern Med* 98:315–319, 1983.

Reisin E, Messerli FH, Ventura HO, et al: Renal haemodynamic studies in obesity hypertension. *J Hypertens* 5:397–400, 1987.

Race

Chrysant SG, Danisa K, Kem DC, et al: Racial differences in pressure, volume and renin interrelationships in essential hypertension. *Hypertension* 1:136–141, 1979.

Dunn FG, Oigman W, Sundgaard-Riise K, et al: Racial differences in cardiac adaptation to essential hypertension determined by echocardiographic indexes. *J Am Coll Cardiol* 1:1348–1351, 1983.

Dustan HP: Does keloid pathogenesis hold the key to understanding black/white differences in hypertension severity. *Hypertension* 1995;26(Part 1):858–862.

Dustan HP: Hypothesis: growth factors and racial differences in severity of hypertension and renal diseases. *Lancet* 1992; 339:1339–1340.

Frohlich ED: State-of-the-Art: Hemodynamic differences in black and white patients with essential hypertension. *Hypertension* 15:675–680, 1990.

Frohlich ED, Messerli FH, Dunn FG, et al: Greater renal vascular involvement in the black patient with essential hypertension. A comparison of systemic and renal hemodynamics in black and white patients. *Mineral Electrolyte Metab* 10:173–177, 1984.

Messerli FH, de Carvalho JGR, Christie B, et al: Essential hypertension in black and white subjects: Hemodynamic findings and fluid volume state. *Am J Med* 67:27–31, 1979.

Women

Gueyffier F, Boutitie F, Boissel JP, et al: for the INDIANA Investigators. Effect of antihypertensive treatment on cardiovascular outcomes in women and men: a meta-analysis of individual patient data from randomized, controlled trials. *Ann Intern Med* 126:761–767, 1997.

Sibai BM: Treatment of hypertension in pregnant women. *N Engl J Med* 335:257–265, 1996.

Wenger NK, Speroff L, Packard B: Cardiovascular health and disease in women. *N Engl J Med.* 329:247–256, 1993.

Woods JW: Oral contraceptives and hypertension. *Hypertension* 11(suppl II):11–15, 1988.

Index

In this index, *italic* page numbers designate figures; page numbers followed by "t" designate tables; *See also* refers to related topics.

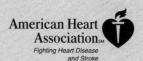
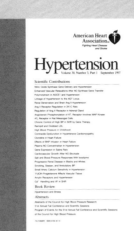